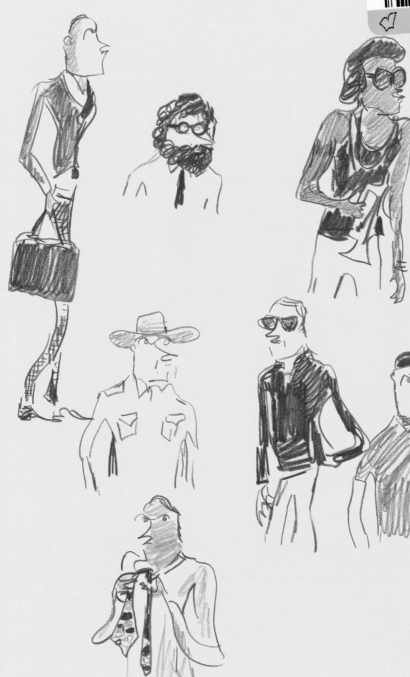

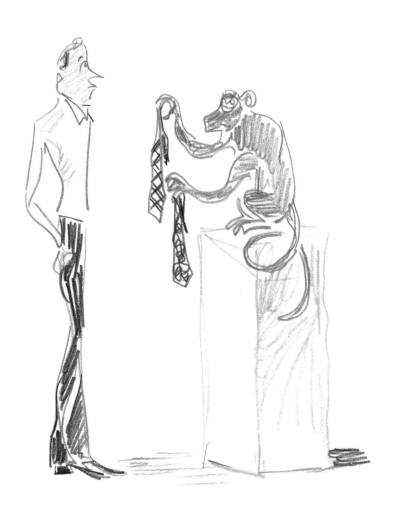

How TO BE A
MAN

by GLENN O'BRIEN

Illustrated by Jean-Philippe Delhomme

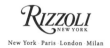

RIZZOLI NEW YORK

New York · Paris · London · Milan

For Gina and Oscar

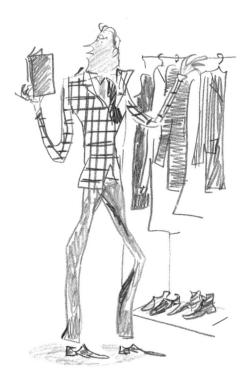

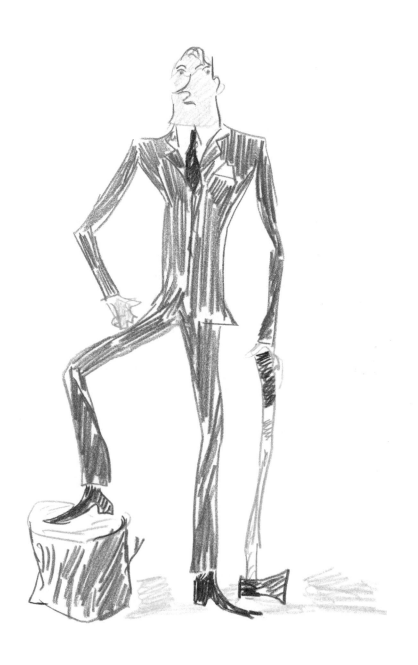

HOW TO BE A MAN

Don't just lie there. Get up and evolve!

Anybody can have a penis, two testicles, and a Y chromosome. You might be a man, technically, but that is not enough anymore. Be a man in full—the full monty. Like the U.S. Army used to tell us, "Be all you can be." Be an army of one. Be an alpha and an omega too. This might be called the human race, but it's also mankind. You, sir, are the crown of creation. So far. Don't blow it.

Manhood is a realm, so you might as well rule it. Use your head. Give it your best shot. Don't take it lying down. Stand up and be counted. Tell it like it is. Let the chips fall where they may. Put your pants on one leg at a time. Tell 'em where they can stick it. No pussyfooting. Give it all you've got. Walk it like you talk it. Put your money where your mouth is. Hit the nail on the head. Stop the buck here. And in the end give 'em something to remember you by.

Socrates said, "Know thyself." Oscar Wilde said, "Be yourself; everyone else is taken." Matthew Arnold said, "Be neither saint nor sophist led, but be a man." Nietzsche said, "Man is something to be surpassed." I say, "What are you waiting for, man?"

Right or wrong, man has always seen himself as special. We've hyped ourselves as reasonable facsimiles of God. But too often, when the going got tough, we've expected a bailout from a presumed creator. Unacceptable!

As Mark Twain pointed out, "Man is the only creature that blushes, or needs to." According to what is supposedly our instruction manual, as the crown of creation man is supposed to have dominion over the earth and its creatures. And while that might not be working out quite as well as expected, all the more reason we should step it up a notch. If God arrives, which I don't expect, looking like a Marine drill instructor a mile high, which I'd like, we want to be able to yell out, "Sir, no excuse, sir!"

Being a man really means being everything a man can be. Evolution is our business. Under the right circumstances and with the right effort a man can be far more than just a man; he can be a gentleman, a sportsman, an inventor, an artist, a philosopher, a bard, a magician, or a hero. Some think he can even be a god, but that's another story.

This is just a collection of musings on how to be a man...better. One step at a time. Forward, or maybe backward, depending on the situation.

The world changes quickly. Man, science informs us, changes slowly. It has taken nature a million years to get us here—ten thousand here to evolve nose hair or ten thousand there to perfect the suntan. It has been a long march to develop the features that will better ensure our survival. But those sophisticated mechanisms so painstakingly developed won't get us out of this one! The jig is up. Now the world is wobbling from our presence. And so now we have to be more and more alert as to how we can adapt ourselves to the facts and manage this ancient organism, with all its flaws and weaknesses, through an ever more challenging environment.

In Homer's time, a single man could know all that men knew as a species. Pretty much, anyway. Kings, chiefs, and priests were the repositories of the collective knowledge and wisdom of the tribe. Heroes conversed with the gods and sometimes schtupped them. The human brain, which, when it failed, was often splattered on the ground by bronze axes, was the only available source of gigabytes. A man was great because he was the fullness of mankind. He knew the names of the stars and distant tribes many days away. When something had no name, he gave it one. He knew the lore of the gods and how to appease them. He knew how to build a house. He knew what herbs would heal a wound or change a mind. He knew how to propitiate the powers of nature, how to propagate crops and livestock, and how to make wine and make war. He knew how to address the people and move them to action. He knew how to dance and that maybe it would even rain afterward.

Today a man can know only a minuscule portion of the sum knowledge of man. Through the exponential expansion of the race, the individual man has been vastly diminished. He knows an iota of what is known. His thoughts and actions may not matter. Are you going to settle for that?

Man has been reduced everywhere, serving the hive like an ant or a bee, toiling away at mechanical tasks and never approaching a knowledge of the whole, or performing the great work. There are no Renaissance men because there is no Renaissance. Or is it the other way around?

Maybe it's time for a change. It's time to reboot. Put up or shut up. Man up, not overboard. Get up. Stand up. Turn the page.

HOW TO BE A GENTLEMAN

Most of us were brought up with some notion of being a gentleman. To a boy, it might sound funny at first, because aren't the ladies supposed to be the gentle ones, while we males are out there sweating and killing, dragging home sides of venison, and clubbing and clawing our way to the ever-shifting top of the evolutionary ladder? But gradually we learn that "gentleman" actually means we should be "gentle" in certain areas, mostly indoors, as in being well mannered and well behaved as opposed to being rough, ill-mannered, and badly behaved. We learn that gentleness will be our cover for being a man, with all the brutal baggage that entails. We will say "please" and "thank you" and "I beg your pardon" and diligently open doors for ladies while remaining alert and prepared to kill communists in far-off countries.

But, in fact, "gentleman" doesn't come from "gentle"; it's the other way around. "Gentle" comes from "gentleman," and "gentleman" comes from "gens," or "race," and it means being of good family, good blood, or top-drawer DNA. And that, of course, means (or meant until recently) belonging to the "right" class and the "right" race. Now, I guess, it means having the "right stuff."

Being gentle once meant that one was entitled to bear arms, an entitlement that is safest when restricted to men of good family. If the gents needed extra help, the peasantry could always pick up a hoe or an axe. The gentleman was the knight, a chivalrous fellow who could show up for war with his own horse, armor, and squire. As far back as the ancient Greeks, the gentleman/chevalier was a fellow who could afford all the trappings of knighthood. During the Middle Ages, the idea of knighthood became associated with the standard of conduct now known as chivalry.

Today chivalry is taken to mean opening the car door for a woman or giving her your arm when she's picking her way over cobblestones in Manolo Blahnik spikes. In short, chivalry is now about making a woman feel like a lady. Modern courtly behavior is seen as descended from the codes of the armed horsemen of the Crusades. But much of their concept of knightly honor was derived from the codes of the knights of Islam—honesty, loyalty, and courtesy were expected from a knight as much as military know-how and the skills of the court. A gentleman knew how to treat a lady, how to use the right fork, how to negotiate a surrender, and how to execute captives politely.

Over centuries, as we became less dependent on cavalry, so being a gentleman became less a matter of bearing arms or of birth and heredity than a matter of "chivalrous instincts and fine feelings." Before I graduated from Georgetown University, which was founded in Washington, D.C., in 1789, a group of us discovered that, as Georgetown students had been declared gentlemen by an Act of Congress, we were entitled to wear swords. Somehow none of us managed to strap them on, perhaps because the local police, sensitized by race riots, arson, and mass antiwar demonstrations in the streets, took a dim view of an armed populace, even armed preppies. But that ancient law did point out that even in a classless society there were mighty ruins of class everywhere, and knowing the words, forms, usages, and possibly the right handshake might win us access to the company of a certain class. The streets might be in flames, but you still don't want anyone ruining your dinner party.

The gentleman observes a code; that code varies somewhat from country to country and region to region. It has evolved over a long time and it includes many trivial and recherché provisions, but observing this code is not a matter of being to the manner or the manor born. Much of the gentlemanly mode can be picked up through attentive apery. It's not, as they say, rocket science. It's more like NASA protocol or the Boy Scout Oath. And though the code has evolved over centuries, it has also devolved considerably. It seems generally agreed upon that we live in one of those decadent "decline and fall" periods, during which great civilizations crumble and the mighty are brought low. In other words, today you will probably be regarded as a gentleman in most places if you don't blow your nose on your sleeve or beat your wife.

Thus it falls to us to hold the line against this historical trend of decline and fall. The barbarians are already inside the gates. We must fill the sandbags of elegance against the rising tide of vulgarity. We must guide the human race onward and upward lest the graph of evolution dip once more toward the mire and cultural oblivion of a Dark Age. And we know what will happen if we don't rise to the challenge. Chaos tends to bring out the law-and-order crowd, and we know how much fun they are.

Being a gentleman is really a matter of being sensitive and observant in all situations and not giving offense as one elevates the tone and terms of transactions. A gentleman is reason personified. He improvises. Nevertheless, a good education in etiquette—even in outmoded and obsolete usages—is a considerable help in mustering up a charming personality. Etiquette gives us precedents, and, if nothing else, it will help you win over ladies and the aged.

It is an excellent tactic to be unfailingly polite. If you are cheerful, solicitous, and appear kind and attentive, you will be welcome almost everywhere. Strangers will believe that you like them. Your enemies will be thwarted, even disarmed by the relentless good vibrations you transmit.

Gentlemanly behavior is the secret key to a utopian society. Marx, Engels, and Lenin preached "the withering away of the state," believing that the state exists only to regulate class conflict. But at this stage of history, statelessness will be achieved not through armed struggle but through culturally enforced codes of manners. I believe that the true anarchist, the exponent of freedom and enemy of intrusive government, must see good manners are the inevitable substitute for laws. A healthy society doesn't need many laws because offensive behavior "just isn't done."

In the mass-media age, traditional concepts of morality have been erased. Today when you say "morals," you mean sex. But sex is just the visible tip of the iceberg that sank the *Titanic* of culture. True morality precludes such vices as covetousness, parsimony, usury, and the good old seven deadlies: wrath, greed, sloth, pride, envy, gluttony, and the too-well-publicized lust. Virtue, the ancient code of *virtus* or manhood, is about far more than keeping it in your pants.

One forgotten sin formerly high on the list is acedia, which sounds like a model of Toyota but means discouragement, apathy, or listlessness. Discouragement should be nipped in the bud by the encouragement of one's fellows, but today it is barely noticed, except as a symptom to be medicated. Undoubtedly there are many among us whose use of selective serotonin reuptake inhibitors could be replaced quite easily by a few well-placed compliments and an atmosphere of cordial community.

Another notion of sin that should be revived by gentlemen and other examiners of conscience is "vainglory," or simply vanity, which is like pride but sillier and more idiotic. Vainglory is probably the sin most committed in today's narcissistic society, except in the Midwest and the South where gluttony may still hold a slight edge.

Sin may seem a tainted concept today, due to the crackpot codes of religious zealots. There seems to be a lot of excess stoning going on in the Middle East, while back in the U.S.A., many Christians believe that it is a sin (1) for a wife not to submit to her husband, (2) to not be content with your wages, (3) to joke, (4) to listen to fables, and (5) to neglect to watch for the imminent return of Jesus Christ. Oh, yeah, and (6) to scoff. I'm guilty of that one all the time.

A gentleman definitely scoffs on occasion. It is one of our best techniques for correcting the unreasonable behavior of others when they don't mind their manners or moral p's and q's. Sin, in religion, is the violation of moral rules. But bad manners constitute a secular notion of the violation of moral rules that needn't be any less thoroughgoing or stringent than that of the religious kind. Manners are generally based on reason, or the common-sense consideration of others. Manners needn't be revealed to us mystically, and they lead to an even better standard of behavior—clarity.

I recommend antique etiquette books to my clients because they provide some perspective on just how far we have fallen from grace. While Emily Post's 1922 book *Etiquette* may not apply today in the entirety of its details (such as her prohibition of a lady sitting to a gentleman's left in a carriage), the spirit of her etiquette is as relevant as ever, and some conventions that are held obsolete today are still relevant.

I'm particularly fond of this proscription: "You must never introduce people to each other in public places unless you are very certain beyond a doubt that the introduction will be agreeable to both. You cannot commit a greater social blunder than to introduce, to a person of position, someone she does not care to know…"

Whatever a gentleman needs to know can usually be picked up by a bright young man who lives by the Golden Rule, generally stated as: do unto others as you would have others do unto you. Details can also be gleaned from etiquette books, and it doesn't hurt to give Aristotle's *Nicomachean Ethics* a good read. It will fill you in on the details of vice and virtue that are no longer part of civility's syllabus.

We live in a rude age in which social life has descended from elegant private balls and intimate dinners to hog-wild corporate blowouts with liquor sponsors, invitation by flowchart title, velvet ropes handled by brutes, guest lists enforced by clipboard-wielding hussies, shameless crashers, step-and-repeat sideshows staged for paparazzi, and open bars until 9:00 p.m. only. The social niceties are of a bygone age. But rather than accepting the ways of the wasteland, we must take these endless slaps at human dignity as the challenge they are and strike back, striving to reintroduce at every opportunity the consciousness and sensitivity required by civilization. Or we must die trying. But we'll fight like the gentlemen of a new age. Our weapons will not be broadsword, mace, and cudgel; they will be wit, satire, mockery, and chiding. Not the longbow but the bon mot.

Tonight I'm gonna party like it's 1599.

HOW TO BE AN ANIMAL

Such natural freedoms are but just: There's something generous in mere lust.
—John Wilmot, 2nd Earl of Rochester, from "A Ramble in St. James' Park"

The job of childhood is to become a better human. The job of adulthood is to become a better animal.

As animals, humans are a little slow. By the time we learn how to walk, lots of species are getting old. This is because humans are very complex and it takes lots of time to grow and program all that equipment.

At first the animal in us has it easy. Breathing, running, eating…all that stuff is kind of a snap. It's the human stuff that's hard, like sitting still in school or long division. Fast-forward a few decades in life and it's the other way around. By the time we navigate the business world and climb the social ladder, our back goes out and we can't read the *Times* without glasses.

As a species, we get caught up in the drama and details of humanity and so are often neglectful of our animal nature and innate skills. Historically, many of man's greatest mistakes have occurred when he has mistook himself for a god or an angel and forgotten that he is also an animal—a mammal, to be specific. And so while philosophy remains a great consolation, there is still meat to be eaten, seed to be sown, and a moon to be howled at.

Of course, you don't have to eat meat to be a man or an animal, although we seem to be the only breed that exercises an option in the matter. I have plenty of friends who do without flesh eating one way or another, and I think that evolution has perhaps taken us in multiple directions. As a member of the Type O blood group, I feel that my cave-man heritage demands that I eat meat regularly to be at my peak. Those of you in the A group may be perfectly content eating spaghetti, chickpeas, spinach, and so on. And you B people will probably want all that and a glass of milk to top it off. This is fine, and you sodbusters should lay off those of us with stalking in our blood. We won't begrudge you your legumes in profusion.

Men are animals plus, but down deep, if we don't keep the old beast happy there will be trouble. This is a very complicated subject, but as an old rooster who admires the spring chicken, I have learned the hard way that physical fitness is of primary importance. This chapter should be a book (hmm), but in the meantime I would like to jot down a few notes here.

We are made to walk. If we do not, we will lose the ability. If you can walk there, do it, not only for the exercise but because that's how a man gets ideas. The rhythm of walking, combined with the concept of moving from point to point, is the perfect context for ideation. I've gotten many of my best ideas on sidewalks and fairways. Musicians and songwriters have often told me that walking is a good mode for picking tunes up out of the firmament.

Do not put yourself in a cage. Naturally getting arrested is a must to avoid, but we are not meant to live in a box or work in a cubicle. It's not worth it. Better to be a traveling salesman or a shepherd. We live amid vicious euphemisms; I have a dictionary that's only thirty-two years old that defines "studio apartment" as an apartment suitable for an artist's studio, being equipped with large windows, high ceilings, etc. A real apartment is a suite of rooms. If you live in a room, you live in a cell. Perhaps it's time that single persons form communes to share the comforts of home—imagine a monastery devoted to, say, mirth rather than religion. It's a thought.

Do not resist the urge to dominate. It's a biological imperative. It's a tough job but somebody's got to do it. Follow me, men!

Getting enough sleep is essential. If God meant us to wake up at a certain time, he would have given our brains an alarm clock. (Oh wait, he did.) Sure you can get by on less sleep, but perchance to dream?

Be fit but not freaky. In ten years or so that gym-created physique will look every bit as stylish as polyester leisure suits. Tumescent muscles not only require too much upkeep, they spoil the line of one's tweeds. The proportions of classical statuary will always be the correct human style.

Appetites are usually right, unless you have damaged them. Disordered appetites are common since man has been alienated from natural environments. Many of the reasons that we see the dead walking among us are to be found on the menu. Artificial sweeteners; "corn sugar" (aka "high-fructose corn syrup" until changed by industry propagandists in September 2010); meat and dairy products poisoned by hormones, unnatural feeds, and confinement-based agriculture; and foods polluted by pesticides and processing: these have created an experimental new human being. He will not survive.

Reproduction is an imperative. Men are hardwired to propagate the species and spread their bloodlines over the earth. Women are wired somewhat differently, and so from time to time we will have to compromise. Men will have to refrain from compulsive trifling, habitual lechery, and flagrant promiscuity. Women will have to forgive us once in a while. And maybe those feral holidays of classical yore are due for revival.

It's OK to be an animal. Just be cage free, organically fed, and ungelded—and come when you're called.

MAN IS A
FUR-BEARING MAMMAL

When I heard that Iran's mullahs had issued a fatwa on spiky male hair-dos and men plucking their eyebrows, I scoffed at this silliness, scratching my head through my Caesar-like coif. But eventually I began to think, stroking my chin bristled to the length popular with the Revolutionary Guard.

I knew this proclamation had nothing to do with the Koran or the word of Allah as received by Muhammad; it was likely justified by the hadith, the arcane code of rulings descended from Arab culture as much as from the wisdom of the Prophet. This ruling is along the same lines as the Persian necktie taboo, a symbolic snub of Western culture. Even Muhammad in all his visionary wisdom could not have foreseen the cravat or the faux hawk. Obviously these dicta were improvised by the mullahs to prevent Farsi youth from resembling Brad Pitt in *Ocean's Eleven*.

Funny thing about the plucking, though, because it's not a rampant practice in the decadent West. It is much more prevalent—though a discreet secret—in men with a tendency toward the unibrow. These are swart fellows of stout follicle—Greeks, Turks, Egyptians, and Iranians more often than Americans or Northern Europeans. I'm sure that there have been certain times and places where a lone supraocular bush was considered beautiful but it is globally unfashionable today. I suspect that the monobrow is most common among Iranians, and "Thou shalt not pluck" is less a matter of Islamic discipline than an affirmation of Persian ethnic pride. If plucking is proscribed, can a nose-job ban be far off? Few nations can boast of such a thriving beak-reduction industry. But the more I thought about the plucking ban, the more I realized that the taboo against plucking is a nondenominational one, shared by conservatives of many cultures.

Grooming phobia has nothing to do with scripture or even oral tradition but is a sort of unspoken code of regular-guyness as widespread in the United States as it is in Iran. Among the masses of the heartland, it is a given that real guys don't pluck—they may eat quiche or drive a Volvo, but they don't slather on depilatories or skulk into waxing salons and electrolysis parlors. They just sprout hair naturally, without intervention, wherever God's providence or fickle chance determines.

Real men do get haircuts and they shave, almost as religiously as Mussulmen, Sikhs, and Hasidim do not. The haircut and the shave are where professedly real men draw the line on grooming. Their brows, chest patches, and back fur grow wild and free, as untended as vacant lots; peculiarly, this is considered the way it should be, as if random hair were integral to God's plan for man and to remove it was a sign of a sinfully feminine vanity.

Some men allow the barber to trim the hair sprouting from ear or nose, but they might hesitate to perform such grooming on themselves. In some cases, particularly among aging men, we see the growth of massive politburo-size brows. No doubt these hedges of hair are driven by that twilight surge of testosterone that also pushes the prostate beyond its customary bounds, and so they are the fruit of the man-sap, as masculine as a gravel voice or steely stubble. And as one of the prime tools in our arsenal of expressions, these bristly plumes enhance a man's ability to silently semaphore suspicion, displeasure, or concentration. "Aren't they magnificent?" one imagines virile sexagenarians purring at the mirror. Hmm.

I recently met a fine fellow with extraordinary brows. He is well spoken and dapper—a scholar and a gentleman. His only quirk is his flaunting of brows of Brezhnevian proportion, immaculately combed upward to startling height and effect. At our first encounter I could barely resist asking what he was thinking about, flaunting these mustache-size plumes? Is it as a form of topiary? Are these brows being groomed for comb-over duty in case of future hairline recession? Are they strange sexual talismans? I couldn't even ask his girlfriend, a longtime friend. I was baffled, dumbstruck. Perhaps on some night when the wine flows freely, I shall dare to inquire: Why? What do you do with them?

This is an extreme and unusual case. Brow pride seems as antiquated today as muttonchops or handlebars. Yet the fact remains that non-scalp, non-beard hair is problematic for the determinedly regular guy. He may be confused by it, or intimidated, as he is by many facets of his appearance. Surely fulsome brow, chest, and back hair is manly, but is there not a line over which it is too much, where it becomes ursine or simian? Why is this growth more sacrosanct than, say, the lawn?

There is clearly too much hair when a man's woman tells him there is. It's ironic that women freely complain about the prominence of a man's secondary sexual characteristics when she wouldn't impugn the primary. "Are we not men?" the too-hairy male must wonder, in Devo-like perplexity. "I am what I am," he thinks, as Popeye once did. He is confused when women adjudge his chest and back hair, the freak flag of his endocrinological majesty, to be too much, unsightly, or even repulsive.

Here are the horns of a dilemma: should he trim or, god forbid, wax, or is that way too gay? The regular guy's instinct is to think of himself as nature and of woman as artifice. But this instinct is inevitably challenged by doubts. Perhaps his hair has begun to desert him as well and he begins to feel the agony of Samson. Or he is graying and suddenly the world sees him differently, though he himself feels as lively as ever. And now he begins to learn the terrible truth. How did William Butler Yeats put it? "That is no country for old men…" Yes, where age was once revered, today it is reviled. Silver is seen as rust. And what is this hair sprouting faster and faster from ears and nose? Where do these eyebrows think they are going?

The man, having spent a lifetime religiously observing regular-guy philosophy, which is not unspoken but mostly codified in boorish jokes, still feels allegiance to that minimally groomed natural man, but he begins to see that the best naturalistic appearance is not natural at all but a carefully calculated pose. It is at this stage that the regular guy undergoes a covert conversion. He begins to dye his hair, probably with something like Just For Men, a man's hair dye, as if men's hair differed from women's, as if use of a product used by women would somehow transform him into a her.

Or perhaps he will capitulate, surrendering grooming decisions to the woman he loves, trusting that she admires his masculinity and will administer it wisely and not pluck his Samsonian virility to within an inch of swish. He will enter the beauty salon by the back door.

The man may even become civilized, clearing away the underbrush at the gateways to his senses. He may, even in Persia, opt for the bicameral brow after all, finding in its symmetry a new reflection of the natural order. He may find a new sense of proportion in the groomed chest thatch, judging it as he would a lawn and learning to mow when propitious, striking that fine balance between dolphin and yeti that is man. No longer will his shirt push away from his breast. No longer will a furry cravat poke through his open collar. No longer will spontaneous talk erupt behind his back at the beach. And possibly he will shave microseconds off his time in the 100-meter butterfly.

Never mind the mullahs or the yahoos! Man must groom to evolve. He must choose the hair nature will provide him in the next life. Pluck away, Persian brothers. May your dual brows arch nobly like those of Michelangelo's *David* (but pluck with professional help lest overplucking cause them to arch like Liza Minnelli's David). Go for a lightly rough line that imitates nature and nothing perfectly geometrical. The well-groomed man will feel sleek and clean and perhaps even more godlike. And hopefully more Apollo-like than, like, Yahweh.

Bears and Bares

I remember that first chest hair. The horror! One single, long, black hair at the periphery of an innocent aureole, like a python beached on a sandy desert island. What was happening to my nipples? It was like watching Jekyll morph into Hyde. I hadn't even figured out why I had nipples. Now that I was twelve, they were going haywire. I had no choice. I found a pair of tweezers and… Ouch!

That wasn't what chest hair was supposed to look like. It wasn't supposed to be all alone. But it wasn't for long. Naturally this act of defiance toward nature opened the hormonal floodgates. I pulled one out and hundreds arrived to replace it. The testosterone flowed like wine, and soon I was furry from nipple to clavicle, and it was good. I felt like a man and had to do manly things to sate that feeling.

In the locker room one learned that there were many states of bodily hairiness, from furry Italians to the smooth, almost feminine Nordics. I felt just about right, somewhere in between. Neither ape nor androgyne, I felt lucky. And it was at just the right time, because chest hair came into fashion in the sixties.

In the early twentieth century men had chest hair, but they tended to hide it under undershirts and two-piece bathing costumes. Hair existed in real life but not in the best of all possible worlds. It was too animalistic and funky. And then, in 1934, Clark Gable removed his shirt in the film *It Happened One Night*, dooming the undershirt to near extinction. It was a very smooth chest that greeted millions of swooning women (and maybe a couple of men).

Even the natural man of legend, Tarzan of the Apes, naturally confined his hair to his head. There is a most amusing photo from the Florida location of the 1941 film *Tarzan's Secret Treasure* showing the star Johnny Weissmuller, the most famous Tarzan of all, with the film's crew; five guys including the producer have gone topless, Tarzan style. Of the six bare-chested fellows only one, Weissmuller, is totally smooth. And so it was with every Tarzan, from Stellan Windrow in 1918, through Elmo Lincoln, Gene Pollar, P. Dempsey Tabler, James H. Pierce, Frank Merrill, Weissmuller, Buster Crabbe, Herman Brix, Glenn Morris, Lex Barker, Gordon Scott,

Denny Miller, Jock Mahoney, Ron Ely (save some slight cleavage shadow), Christopher Lambert, Miles O'Keeffe, and Casper Van Dien. In the entire history of the franchise, only Mike Henry, who played Tarzan from 1966 to 1968 and Clint Walker, who played him in a silly B picture, had chest hair. None had beards. (There must have been razors in the wreckage of the plane.) I guess that made it easier to tell Tarzan from the apes, but it's strange, all the same. Maybe Lord Greystoke figured out how to wax his chest from the bees during all that jungle downtime.

This hairless ideal prevailed among the stars of gladiator movies and biblical epics in the CinemaScope fifties and sixties. Steve Reeves, who went from Mr. America, Mr. World, and Mr. Universe to playing Hercules, Goliath, Romulus, Aeneas, and other larger-than-life characters, was one of the first film stars to popularize the hairless bodybuilder aesthetic. Top bodybuilders have always been into depilation. Body hair and oil don't mix. Even filmic he-men like Victor Mature dared only show a sort of five o'clock shadow between the pecs. Few boxers sported chest hair; even the great Italians like Primo Carnera and Rocky Marciano were sparsely sprouted.

Hairy chests on men only came in with the intellectual movement toward naturalism and realism. A new breed of actors arrived on the scene who showed that real men realistically depicted had some hair under their shirts—Marlon Brando, Steve McQueen, and Lee Marvin. Even the supersmooth Paul Newman had hair sprouting around his nipples, sort of the way I did at thirteen.

As the sixties progressed, they brought more natural attitudes—first with sexually confident cool guys and then with the atavistic, back-to-nature hippies. Hippie chicks were sprouting underarm hair and fuzzy legs. All things natural suddenly seemed, well, natural. And this news was being broken to the public by guys like Sean Connery (whose hirsute chest as 007 is celebrated by Austin Powers's barbigerous bosom), James Garner, Burt Reynolds, Tom Jones, and Jim Brown (he of the first famous chest-fro). By the early eighties, body hair was a requisite of manliness. But it was not something manly men thought about, or at least talked about, even if their polyester shirts puffed out in front.

When John Travolta danced his way into the hearts of millions as Tony Manero, he did it with his shirt unbuttoned practically to the navel, revealing a briar patch so dark it almost served as an ascot. The hairy chest was very disco, but it was also rock and roll, flaunted by the likes of Gary Glitter, AC/DC, Robert Plant, Gene Simmons, and even the Godfather of Soul, James Brown.

But then in the eighties, something happened. Suddenly hairless pecs as sleek as the marble thorax of Michelangelo's *David* were all the rage. Why? Was it the six-packs of Studio 54's topless bartenders? Was it Iggy Pop, gyrating bare-chested across stages to Marshall-amped power chords? Or was it Calvin Klein? The handsome Calvin appeared in his own ads, bare and sweaty in a Georgia O'Keeffe adobe, as smooth as a Greek god. It was a new look, spreading from the beaches of Fire Island to the streets of the West Village. Or maybe it was the influence of Olympic sensation diver Greg Louganis, whose supple torso thrilled millions. Whatever it was, hair was suddenly disappearing again from the chests of men everywhere. It seemed to start with the gays and then spread through locker-room contact to the straights. Soon entire gymnasiums were as clean as a swim team. But what did it mean?

Superficially it seemed to be about a boy. About boyness. About the Greek ideal of the *eromenos*. (Yeah, you won't see much chest hair on the Spartans of *300*.) The waxing of the chest could only mean one thing. And that is that it's better to be a boy than to be a man. Youth is the ideal! Other boys check you out. You're always first in line. Nothing stands in your way when you're a boy.

But you can't be a boy forever. And if you try to be, you might wind up looking like an old lady instead. So these manly hairs pose a dilemma. Is the chest just another beard, or is it something more essential and closer to the heart?

There are clues. According to a *China Times* article, a London insurance firm, Creechurch Underwriting, has been asked to draw up a policy protecting a certain film star against loss of his chest hair. In 2004 it was reported that Orlando Bloom wore a chest wig for his role in Ridley Scott's *Kingdom of Heaven*. An unnamed source was quoted as saying: "His chest rug is probably the best special effect in the picture."

Today there are two schools of thought. We see very hairy men who let it all hang out, like Robin Williams: "Monkeys [in the zoo] shout I'm in *here* and *you're* walking around like *that?*" And then we see ultra-groomed men like Marilyn Manson for whom the very idea of body hair is simply unimaginable.

It's a mystery. Will evolution eventually banish the body's hair as we move on a smooth trajectory toward the total depilation of the alien "gray," or will these vestiges perhaps gain a new testosterone-fueled momentum, returning us to the jungles from which we swung on vines? It's way too soon to tell. All I know is that before I head for St. Barth's, I'm going to get out the scissors and crop that gray pelt of tit fur down to a half an inch of sheer civilized manliness.

The Rear View

Years ago I accepted an assignment from *Allure*, the beauty magazine, to go for a waxing. I never thought of myself as needing it, but I had been told that I was getting hairy on the back. Like the ears and the nose, the back can get hairier and hairier the longer we persist on earth.

Well, I went to a fancy salon and submitted to the hot wax and it hurt. It wasn't quite like the "Is it safe?" scene in *Marathon Man*, but it hurt like heck. I was gritting and growling. And when it was over the lady asked me if I wanted my ears done and I said no very quickly. Maybe I should have said yes, because the amazing thing is that the back hair never really came back.

And truth be told there were times on the beach when I've seen certain friends, the famous painter, the downtown filmmaker, and thought, how the hell can they go around with a back like an orangutan's? Well, today those men are as smooth as I am. Maybe I did that!

And Further Down

We can usually tell what decade a porn picture is from by the hairstyle of the bush. In my youth, women had big bushes. Then came bikini waxes. Next came topiary trimming. Not long ago, the fad was a pubic Hitler mustache. Finally there's the total shave.

I am not a fan of the shave, for woman or for man. I know some people think it's sleek and clean, but it's also infantile. How can there not be some pedophilic angle to this? Nubility is something to be proud of, but it's also something to be managed.

HAIR TODAY
(GONE TOMORROW?)

It's nice to have a good, full, thick head of hair. It keeps you warm. Girls can run their fingers through it. It can be styled into a sculpture. With enough hair, you can wave it like a flag in a heavy-metal frenzy, dishevel it into a "Let's sack Rome" look, or twist it up into the crown of the Rasta man. If it's kinky you can comb it up in an Afro that will scare whitey, even if you're Jewish. It can be the crowning touch of a retro look—from the patent-leather hair of Fred Astaire to a rock-and-roll rooster à la Keith Richards or Johnny Thunders. Styled artfully, a man's hair provides clues to his attitudes. But fortunately for a considerable segment of the male gender, perhaps approaching half of adult males in America, a full head of hair is no longer absolutely necessary for self-respect or acquisition of a love interest.

Male-pattern baldness is bigger than the Republican Party. Midfrontal loss affects one out of four men twenty and over, and two out of three men sixty and over. It's actually a sex hormone that causes baldness, if that's any consolation, the same relentless secretion that makes one's prostate grow to the size of an orange. Baldness isn't about not enough sexual juice but too much. But why are men designed to degenerate in this way from their youthful glory? Is God bald? Some scientists theorize that baldness is an evolutionary development signaling maturity, hence an inclination toward nurturing and a disinclination toward aggression and risk taking. So while baldness might not get you laid, it might get you married.

Still, hair was considered so important through most of the twentieth century that men often resorted to toupees or hairpieces—sometimes illfitting to the point of outlandishness—in an attempt to disguise their male-pattern baldness, as there was a definite cultural bias against men who experienced hair loss. Or they went through painful surgical procedures, such as weaving and grafting. A friend of mine, desperate to stop the erosion of his hairline, employed a stern German Frau with a possible Nazi history to yank on each individual hair to stimulate growth at the follicle. I suppose there have been successful exceptions, but I think that generally wigs really work only when they are acknowledged as wigs, as in the case of Andy Warhol, or back in the powdered-wig days (a time of endemic lice), when heads were shaved or shorn and luxuriant locks were donned like hats, à la Johnny Depp in *The Libertine*.

The toupee is really a trompe l'oeil hat. Some men have pulled it off as natural hair, but most rug wearers, even celebrities with vast resources, have failed miserably. (Marv Albert, Howard Cosell, Trent Lott, Charlton Heston, Frank Sinatra, and Bud Selig come to mind.) Still our cultural prejudices dictate that male-pattern baldness is not the best look, and given the choice between a lout with locks and a mensch with androgenic alopecia, a lot of potential mates might make the wrong choice. Pattern baldness isn't cool. But total baldness now seems to be another story. A savior of the bald arrived in the person of Michael Jordan, who epitomized superhuman physical achievement and confident alpha sexuality—and all without a hair on his head. Well, there were actually a bunch of saviors. Yul Brynner had achieved stardom and sex symbol-dom when he shaved his head for the lead role of the king in *The King and I* in 1956, and Telly Savalas went entirely hairless as the hard-boiled titular character in *Kojak* in the seventies. Despite his resemblance to the Bond villain he also played, Ernst Stavro Blofeld, Savalas was considered in the "sexiest man alive" league by many women. But somehow it was Jordan's allover shave that set off the wave of stars with shaved heads—including many top athletes and performers like Isaac Hayes, Bruce Willis, Billy Corgan, Vin Diesel, Michael Stipe, Billy Zane, Ving Rhames, and Captain Jean-Luc Picard. The shaved head is the ultimate in minimalism, and no other hairstyle offers such timelessness.

Worse than all but the worst toupees is the comb-over, a tactic by which a man attempts to cover his bald areas with strands of hair diverted from the back and sides. Making hair look naturally plentiful by artful combing is not easy. (In fact a father and son in Orlando, Florida, were actually granted U.S. Patent 4,022,227 in 1977 for their combing technique.) Of course the comb-over may forestall the appearance of baldness, but it's often a stopgap measure carried on for too long in a losing cause. Particularly egregious examples of the comb-over have been perpetrated by Rudolph Giuliani, General David Petraeus, John McCain, Sam Donaldson, and Donald Trump. The latter's hair seems to be a miracle of engineering that transcends the term "comb-over"—it's more of a cantilever-over. My friend Jean-Paul Goude, who resurrected his own hair through hard work and cutting-edge medical treatment after spending years in a base-ball cap, refers to the comb-over as "moving the suburbs to Paris." Alas, the suburbs will never be mistaken for the first arrondissement. In Japan, comb-over wearers are kiddingly called "bar-code men" for their striated scalps.

Baldness finally found its miracle drug in 1992 when finasteride, a drug intended to treat enlarged prostates, was approved by the FDA for treating baldness. (It is marketed under the names Propecia and Proscar.) Finasteride works by altering the hormonal mix that makes baldness kick in, and it does indeed regrow hair for most of the men who try it. But hormones are tricky things to mess with, and the possible side effects of the drug include impotence, erectile dysfunction, abnormal ejaculation, and gynecomastia. Which leads us to the question: why grow hair to attract women if you can't have proper sex with them, or if you wind up looking more like them? Furthermore, a Swedish regulatory agency concluded that erectile dysfunction caused by Propecia may persist after use of the drug is discontinued.

Hair transplanting (also called "plugs") is the medical version of the comb-over, in which hair is moved from one place to another. Obviously success with this procedure is based on having enough hair to move. Transplants are also painful and can cause scarring, and not all men are good prospects. Some years ago we saw NBA coach (now TV analyst) Jeff Van Gundy getting plugged publicly, and it was not a pretty sight. He looked much better when he abandoned the idea. He suddenly looked honest.

Like many men, the author is not a good candidate for a head shave, having a cranial dent that seems to have resulted from an intoxicated obstetrician with forceps as well as a purple birthmark resembling a Rorschach inkblot. Fortunately his hair seems to be holding up. An alternative to the shave is the short-buzz strategy, used effectively by patchy fellows like Ed Harris and John Malkovich. Then there is the Lenin look, in which prominent facial hair distracts from the dome's dearth. The most important thing to consider regarding male-pattern baldness is that no one is as concerned with hair loss as the hair loser. If you're worried about hairline recession impacting your attractiveness, make more money and be funnier. No one has gotten laid more than Jack Nicholson, whose hairline has receded steadily as his fame has advanced.

A few words of advice: if you shave your head, wear hats in winter and sunscreen when it's sunny. A model-agency exec who looks after a tribe of youthful male models, some of whom shave their heads, told me about a razor designed specifically for that purpose called the HeadBlade. You slip it on your finger like a ring and stroke your scalp. It gives a clean, close shave in less time than conventional razors.

A completely shaved head is a proud head. It's an attention getter, so the proprietor of a newly shaved head should make sure that his wardrobe is up to par. Sometimes a man who is trying to hide something dresses schlumpily, hoping, consciously or not, to fade into the background. To go proudly chrome domed, dress with verve lest cool be taken for chemo.

If you do not choose to go all the way, as a rule, the shorter the hair, the less obvious the hair loss. I have worn my hair cropped short for years, and although I haven't lost any hair, I have noticed that all of my balding friends who have adopted this style look younger and less conspicuously balding.

Gray Liberation

I went gray young. Then one salt-and-pepper summer, I grew my hair long and a woman friend informed me that I was much too young and handsome to have all that gray in my hair. So I dyed it my natural color.

I used Clairol, as I recall. The women's kind. I think I even knew the model on the cover of the box. I find hair dyes marketed to men silly, at the very least, and possibly even insidious. What are they trying to tell us? Hair is hair. By marketing to men, they are telling us that using this product will not chemically transgender us. The same strategy of feeding on insecurity is used to market many products that are needlessly assigned a gender, like men's deodorants or women's cigarettes.

Anyway, I looked good brunette. Probably younger. Then one day, I couldn't find the usual shade of brown and tried another brand. My hair came out much darker. The next day, I walked into an office where I made regular appearances and was greeted by a chorus of laughter. I never dyed again, and occasionally I wonder, What was I thinking? Of course I was buckling to cultural prejudice. Men are easily seduced into covering the gray out of fear of aging, and it works fine at first—sounds like drugs, right?—but as men get older the whole proposition gets shakier. Why doesn't he have any gray? What is he going to do? Keep coloring into the old folks' home or go gray overnight announcing that he had a terrible shock? Dyeing your hair is like going to war; you need to go into it with an exit strategy.

We live in an era of ageism that ranges in degree from the ridiculous to the creepy. The venerable has given way to the venereal. Young now gets the honors that once belonged to old. I guess it's the punk legacy—live fast, die young, and leave a good-looking corpse. That works out well for one's heirs, but it's not a course I endorse. I say live long, date young, and leave a good-looking empire.

So let those millions of men try to chase away that gray with their men's-only concoctions. I'm proud of my white hairs. I earned them, and they look really good, I think, as long as I have a tan. Rule number one for white hair: if you're not already dark of complexion, get a tan. You'll notice that the lack of contrast between white hair and a white face tends to make one disappear in photographs. This is not good. Look at Giorgio Armani and Ralph Lauren. They know what they're doing by setting off their snowy locks with skin of bronze or gold. And how good does Ted Danson look in his snowy crew cut? Marvelous!

Rule number two: forget about long hair. The only person who ever looked good with long, gray hair was Leon Russell, and now he looks a bit like the abominable snowman. Leon pulled this off in part because he had a young face and dark eyebrows. Dark eyebrows are very important, and even if you are otherwise all natural, I recommend you find a holistic colorist to ensure that your eyebrows remain dark and you remain in the picture.

In a wise world, in an ideal world, age is honored and respected, especially when it is marked by accomplishment, distinction, and wisdom. You are a tribal elder. You've got the know-how. You've got the chops. You've got seniority. You can do things the whippersnappers can't: you can be majestic, esteemed, revered. Venerated can get you laid. Don't dishonor your silver. Cherish it. You earned it. You've got patina, baby! Use it.

BARBER VS. SALON

I think it was the great *Esquire* editor Harold Hayes who said, "A man should not look like he has a haircut or needs one."

Today, as on many occasions, the author needs a haircut. I've been putting it off. It sounds easy, getting a haircut, but it's not so simple. It's hard, in fact. It used to be easy for men to deal with their hair; they simply went to a barber and the barber took care of it. Directions? If the customer were a regular, the barber would say "The usual?" The customer would nod or grunt or say, "Just give me a trim," meaning a little less off. If the customer was a stranger, he might instruct the barber "Give me a regular haircut." Or "Take a little off the top," or "Clean up the back."

Then, in the sixties and seventies, the cultural revolution struck the male hair trade with a sweeping change of perception. Cops and cowboys and hard hats—motivated by jealousy of the seductive prowess of the hirsute British Invasion and the charm for the fair sex demonstrated by local hippie ne'er-do-wells—began growing long, luxuriant, sissy hair. It was soon established that men needed to go to hairdressers and pay five times more to get a hairstyle than they paid to get a haircut. Suddenly guys were going to salons where the walls were covered with magazine photos of John Travolta, Robert Redford, Andy Gibb, Joe Namath, and Al Pacino, and getting shampoos and having blow-dryers pointed at them. Even regular women's hairdressers were going bisexual (their salons, that is). Suddenly your wife's guy, Mr. Dick, was blowing you...out.

Before salons, barbershops didn't have pictures all over the walls because nearly all men got the regular man's haircut. The neighborhood barbershop offered only a little more choice than the one at Parris Island. But at the salon, pictures became necessary, because suddenly a man had to describe what he wanted, and how do you describe what you might not even know? Men were not trained to envision themselves transformed and certainly not trained to instruct a *coiffeur*. Men really wanted someone to just do it, figure out how they should look and make it so. But instead of the painless "take a little off the top," it was now "Give me a Barry Gibb." Or a Tom Jones, or a John Denver. Today we have boys asking for Biebers—back then we had Herman's Hermits.

In the post-barber age, stylists became artists. The new salon was not the barbershop of our youth. No more red, white, and blue pole standing for venous blood, arterial blood, and bandages. No more hot towels and straight-razor shaves. No more cigar smoke and racy periodicals. Truth be told, the men's salon was more like the beauty salon our moms had dragged us into, with its strange dryers and Bride-of-Frankenstein permanent-wave machines and exotic chemical smells.

I hated the whole salon experience. It wasn't that I was uncomfortable in the less traditional atmosphere, but there was an attitude problem. I didn't want to put myself in the hands of an artist, like a blank canvas ready to be transformed by genius. I went to a stylist who wanted to make me look like Morrissey. Another seemed to think I should look like I was in A Flock of Seagulls. I just couldn't find the right hairstylist. Then I went to a Japanese stylist who didn't speak any English, and I had to communicate with him in sign language. That was a little better. Then I went to a guy who was exactly like the Zohan (except that he didn't come on to me), but I came out a different person after every cut. Then for a few years I went to a hairdresser who really thought she was an artist, a fine artist, which had apparently rubbed off on her from cutting a lot of artists' hair. She cut lots of big musicians' hair too, but for some reason she never cut a single. She had accumulated a pretty good art collection in trade, but the downside was that cutting artists' hair had magically made her an artist too. For her first show (in the salon), she dated men she met through classified ads, secretly recording and photographing them. I should have known right then not to trust her with my hair, but it looked pretty good. Then she started telling me that I should drink a particular tea with fiber in it and get high colonics, and then she told me that what I really needed was to get an inner life. In fact, all I needed was a haircut.

I don't know why I went back after that, but then her art career really did start to interfere with the haircutting. I found out that she had been collecting my hair cuttings along with those of other clients. She had Baggies full of famous hair. I freaked and never went back. I mean, I could see her keeping a lock of the Boss's hair, but mine? It was way too voodoo. I still had no inner life. So I decided to cut my own hair.

I think that ideally a man should know how to cut hair. It's one of the basic skills, like shaving, doing the sidestroke, giving artificial respiration, poaching an egg, and applying the Heimlich. I learned to cut hair from observing my friend, the great womanizing hairdresser. I watched how he did it. It was really physical, like massage or Ping-Pong. It was about feel. And I had decided I wanted to look the same every day, so almost every day I cut my hair a little bit. I found that a sort of meditation. It wasn't really about vanity; it was more akin to sculpture and self-awareness.

Even today I'll sometimes go off seeing my regular barber and cut it myself for a while. I think every man should try this as a way of discovering what he really looks like from all angles. But maybe when he's on vacation, in case he really fucks up.

Hair is personal. It has secrets. They say that magicians can kill you with your hair, or at least they think they can, and scientists can clone you with it or tell if you're on dope or if you have heavy-metal poisoning, so to trust someone with your hair means that you are at their mercy, at least symbolically. I am still carrying around a passport in which I have a genuine platinum-blond crew cut. This is the result of me allowing someone close to me to put dark highlights into my salt-and-pepper hair. When I got a considerably shorter haircut, what had previously looked like highlights now looked like a graffiti artist had tagged my head. The salon's solution? Bleach it out. They tried. The tag was still there, but I became a platinum blond. I looked like an older, less muscular version of Robert Shaw in *From Russia with Love*. Hair maintenance shouldn't be such hard work. It should be a pleasure.

When you're a kid, going to the barber is a cool rite of passage—the first manly thing you do. As a boy, I loved getting a haircut. I loved the paper they wrapped around your neck and the cloth they threw over your clothes and the smells and all the mysterious bottles of tonics and creams. I loved getting spritzed on the scalp with witch hazel and whopped with a spray of talc on the neck. I loved the Italian barbers I patronized who kept canaries and would break into song themselves, snatches of opera, and they knew how to make thunder shaking a towel. I remember barber poles that twirled, and I remember hearing for the first time that the red and white stood for blood and bandages, apparently because once upon a time barbers were also the doctors and you'd go to them to have leeches applied for bloodletting.

It was a manly place. All around were guys dozing under hot towels and guys being shaved with deadly looking straight razors. It was a real initiation into manhood. It's hard to believe that the barbershop as we knew it almost disappeared. But it didn't, and happily the old-school barbershop is making a comeback as a retro and charmingly authentic-esque alternative to men's salons. Today's salons masquerade as men's clubs to bring in the patrons, with pool tables and bars decked with arcane bottles of single malt Scotch, but there's a nice simplicity to ye olde barbershop and its lower tab. The barber-style cut is back, but the salon-style do is still with us too. We are now able to select from any hairstyle in history. A man can wear a crew cut, an Oscar Wilde pageboy, an oily pompadour, a Mohawk, a faux hawk, a Jeff Beck shag, or punk spikes, all with surprisingly little cultural meaning. It doesn't mean gay or straight, left or right wing; it doesn't mean anything more than, say, what a shoe means or a shirt. It is not a cultural identifier but a fashion look that can be put on or taken off.

These days I patronize a barber in a large middle-class shop. My man is a Sicilian in his late sixties. I never give out his name, because he doesn't take appointments and often I have to wait for him to do four or five heads before I get my turn. That's because he's really good. There are few places on this planet where they teach barbering the old-fashioned way, and for the Italians barbering is a venerable craft.

But then in July I may go in for a haircut and not pay attention, and when he's finishing up I say, "Hey, why so short?" And then he says, "I'm going on vacation for August!" So I usually wind up cutting it myself for a while and then I'm afraid to go back because he'll complain, "Why you a-do this? Look-a, you ruin da hair!" Sometimes I do get a bit choppy and it's tough for him to repair the damage I've done.

If I'm traveling and I have to go to an unfamiliar barber I usually say, "I want to look like a Roman emperor." Some barbers get that. Or, "You know, a Caesar." It would be great if a discussion of Claudian dynasty hairstyles resulted, but no barber ever asked me what emperor I wanted to look like. I don't want to look like Nero, Otho, or Hadrian, with all that curling-iron work. Julius wore a toupee. Trajan looked like Moe from the Stooges.

I want your basic, simple Augustus. I don't want to look like a Greek fop like Marcus Aurelius. (Ever notice how legendary basketball star Larry Byrd looks like Tiberius? I thought not.) Anyway, if that doesn't work I try "Russell Crowe in *Gladiator*" or "Give me a George Clooney." I think the best look is, as Andy Warhol said, "a good plain look." But you can't ask for that.

Funny but I just saw a picture of me taken by Andy Warhol, circa '72, when I had really long hair. I looked great. Young men should have long hair, because they won't be able to wear it when they're fifty. If you don't believe me, look at Aerosmith. Russell Brand has got about three years left. (No, I just saw *Arthur*. He's done.)

Anyway, I'm going to go face the music now and let the barber yell at me. He hasn't seen me in three months. He's going to be pissed at how I chopped my hair up. But I can't go on like this another day: I'm going to get a haircut.

HOW TO BE SEXUAL

Most men are sexually attracted to women. Don't worry. Having sex with women is natural and most of us manage to pull it off eventually. The trick is simply to find ways to have intercourse with women (in the various senses) without giving them undue power or influence over you. The idea is to remain a man.

There are, of course, vast cultural and social mechanisms that govern relations between the genders, and these will try to push you around for sure, but the prevailing climate ought not be construed or accepted as good, fair, or reasonable. Marriage is like "the house" in Las Vegas, rigged slightly against you and hard to beat in the long run but fun to play against nevertheless.

Somehow, when things go badly, the law tends to take the side of the woman, as do other women and not a few men. As the so-called second sex, woman fiercely defends her role as underdog, lording it over men, while enjoying many advantages and favorable odds. For example, women often position themselves as an aggrieved minority group, even though in the United States they outnumber men by more than four million persons. Relations between men and women have to deal with fictions as well as facts. This means that in dealing with women, a man must always be ready to improvise. Subterfuge may occasionally prove the wisest course—not to give you an unfair advantage in a contest of wills but to allow for peace and the greater good.

You can't count on customs and manners to get you through. Just because things were always done a certain way doesn't mean they will always be done that way. Times change quickly. A few generations back, women were denied the vote; today they govern great nations. Woman is evolving, perhaps faster than we are. It is my theory that women are more suited to life in the densely populated corporate world than men. They are less territorial. They are less subject to the cardiovascular stress that moving through a corporate flowchart induces. They are born collaborators rather than competitors. They seem to handle unnatural environments better than men, perhaps because they carry nature within themselves. And ultimately they are more durable. They will outlast you every time. So a man sometimes needs to look for an edge and use his wits. If you can think of a better way to deal with women, why not try it? Maybe you'll hit on something. Just not her.

Women are essentially different from men, which is why we call relations between the genders *hetero*sexual. Humans are a heterogeneous species. Therefore in sexual relations, heterosexuals are never quite sure what the other person is feeling and can only guess, unlike homosexuals, who can closely identify with their partners. Our partners are a completely different gender with a different physicality and psychology. Some would call women a different species or life form altogether. Are they a superior life form? It depends on who you listen to, but a case could certainly be made that their gender is running the planet behind the scenes and, increasingly, in front of them.

The first step in being a successful heterosexual is to admit it. Admit that you are attracted to women and you are not ashamed of that, even though you don't understand them. You are drawn to women even though your encounters with them have left you baffled, perplexed, humbled, and even slightly damaged. There, don't you feel better already? Why we are attracted to women is something we will discover later on in the process. At first attraction may seem an entirely physical sensation, and for some men it is very specific. Some men even prefer certain parts of the woman to the whole, like a person shopping for chicken parts. I'm a breast man. I'm a leg man. This is a bad road to go down, for it always seems to end up with leftovers. We have to love women holistically, embracing all that they are, the good and the bad, the beautiful and the ugly, the delightful and the terrifying. Women are like medicinal herbs: you may think you have isolated their active ingredient, but all of those other elements are there for a reason.

A lot of it is about sex. That's how our involvement with women gets started. The little head gives the big head ideas. We experience compulsions to mate with them. They notice our attraction and things get complicated. The woman may show a similar interest, but it is not an identical interest, to be sure. And even though we wind up in the most intimate collaboration possible, we are never quite sure of our partner's motivations or rewards. They are mysterious and inscrutable.

Whether men or women enjoy sex more has been the subject of debate for millennia. Even the gods argued about it, and according to Ovid's *Metamorphoses*, in a dispute on the matter between Jupiter and Juno, Tiresias was called upon as an authority since he was a man who'd become a woman and then a man again. (His transformation to a woman occurred after he'd struck two mating snakes.) Tiresias replied, "Of ten parts a man enjoys one only." I know this may seem not only unfair but also hard to believe, and we may fairly conclude that not all women experience sex with equal gusto. But this is handy information to pass along if a woman complains that you are not holding up your end in satisfying her. Tell her that she must be joking, since women enjoy sex ten times more than men do. If you're only getting her off halfway, she's still ahead five to one.

If a relationship gets off to a poor start sexually, forget about it. It probably won't get any better. With exceptions, I have never believed that particular people are "good in bed," the way you might be good at tennis or golf. It is obviously true that some have more interest and some certainly try harder, but the crucial factor is chemistry and fit. A woman might be lousy in bed with John Doe but great in bed with Dick Doe. That's why they call it a sexual relationship and not a sexual contest.

A good indicator of one's prospects with a woman is meeting her mother. Often this provides a fair prognosis of what the younger woman will be like in twenty-some years. If the mother is still attractive and pleasant, your relationship may have a better chance of enduring. Inspect the mother carefully for cellulite, bunions, alcoholism, and widowhood.

Don't let women convert you to their way of thinking about your gender. Don't listen to all that talk about testosterone. If feminists start giving it to you, come right back with your own crackpot theory about estrogen. Testosterone does not cause wars or crime. It makes your ears and nose hairy and your prostate end up the size of a polo ball. Estrogen makes your sleep patterns bad and your memory good. But if they tell you that testosterone is the cause of war, try telling them that estrogen is causing the hole in the ozone layer. Maybe the combined hot flashes of the baby boomers going menopausal are contributing to global warming!

Women tend to be confused about masculinity and femininity. They want men, but they are often unsure how manly they want their men. Some want their man to look like the leader of the pack and act like a puppy. Some just want a puppy, possibly neutered. It's important that we don't fall victim to clichés about sexual roles. Sometimes the best way to attract women is through a deliberate suppression of typical masculine characteristics.

Consider the enormous appeal that gay men have for straight women. When you've lived in New York you're used to hearing from women, "Why are all the great single men gay?" Well, this never was true. And it's even less true today, now that a lot of the great single men have married one another. But the fact is that there are a lot of things that women like about gay men. Gay men aren't threatening to women. They are sympathetic, and they make good advisers for women in love because they know more about men than women do. In general, they think a woman's breasts are fine just the way they are. Gay men have no particular reason to lie to women, unless it's to spare their feelings about their new hairdo or what they're wearing. And they won't criticize them for spending a lot on clothes and their appearance. Straight women love gay men to the extent that they may even try to convert them. An amusing case is the *Seinfeld* episode in which Elaine tries to recruit one "over to our team," despite Jerry's warnings that it's virtually impossible because "they like their own team's equipment."

The girls on *Sex and the City* sleep with typical hetero men and suffer from complex hang-ups because of the usual misunderstandings, but socially they prefer the company of gay men. This situation was not invented by that series's creator and writer, Darren Star. Anyone familiar with anthropology knows that in societies where homosexuality is tolerated, as in many American Indian tribes, heterosexual women often show an enthusiasm for their company. Yes, even the ancient Mayans probably had fag hags. Perhaps in the interest of evolution, or at least more peaceful relationships, we must learn to be gayer heterosexuals.

Do you know what the word "gay" means, soldier? It means "full of or disposed to joy and mirth"! It means lighthearted, exuberantly cheerful, sportive, and merry. It means offhand, for God's sake! In the sixteenth century it meant brilliant, attractive, excellent, fine! So maybe straight men need to be more gay in the old sense of the word. So let's explore the benefits of feigning disinterest in a woman. Let us comport ourselves with good breeding and exquisite manners up to the brink of effeminacy when necessary. Because, men, when the going gets tough, the tough give each other a big hug.

The greatest womanizer I ever knew was a hairdresser, which you might consider being a heterosexual in a homosexual profession. He was the *Shampoo* character come to real life. As with the film's George, his profession was the perfect cover. He was not suspected of being a master womanizer, even though he was surrounded by beautiful models, beautiful rich ladies, and beautiful receptionists. Visiting him at work was like going shopping for girls.

Sexual identities are constructs, and one of the interesting cultural changes in my lifetime has been the disappearance of signifiers between heterosexuals and homosexuals. Liberation and acceptance have made the traditional "out" gay personality almost an endangered species. Some might see this change as a triumph over stereotyping, but at what cost? Some of the most delightful elements of culture have come out of communities of oppressed minorities. "Gay Is the New Black," reads a contemporary T-shirt. Both gays and blacks developed a language to speak to one another and modes of humor and performance that have enriched the larger culture. A lot of blacks aren't very black anymore and a lot of gay people aren't very gay. "Gay" was always a questionable choice of words, but now it can be positively ironic when referring to some lesbian storm troopers and dour double-husband-marrieds. Don't we miss some of the culture of the closet—the subtlety, the refinement, the innuendo?

As the closet has been inhabited less and less, an interesting aspect of the liberation process is how gay identities have evolved in an accepting world. Young gays seem somehow straighter. It's almost as if you can't tell the gays from the straights without a program.

"The gaydar is malfunctioning, Captain!"

"What do you mean, sailor?"

"It's not picking anything up. We can't tell the queers from the straights."

"Should we ask?"

"We can't, Captain. We can't ask or tell!"[1]

Gay culture evolved its own language and codes within a context of hostility and opposition. What happens when the opposition and hostility are gone? Liberation is a great thing, but does this mean that drag queens are an endangered species? Will the leather bar vanish? (Further?) Will the Broadway musical lose its historians? And those archetypes celebrated by The Village People, will they vanish into little-read history? I feel a certain nostalgia for old queer identities and the various "boys in the band." I miss the extreme cultivated mannerism of sissies and the venom of archly droll fairies. Perhaps there are things that are acquired in a closet or a ghetto that are worth holding on to. Do we want to live in a world without fairies and sissies, bitches and drag queens? Do we, Mary?

I don't miss discrimination but I did like the way Andy Warhol used to put it: "I think he's got a problem." But what Andy didn't realize was that being straight can be a problem too. When you think about it, when it comes to sex, just about everybody has a problem. But one man's problem is another man's opportunity.

Like heterosexuality, homosexuality is not really an option. Well, I suppose either is, if you're drunk enough. But it would seem that our interests and options are fairly (although sometimes unfairly) predetermined, or at least the deck we play with is stacked. Science seems to be showing that sexual inclinations are inborn, or at least they are present in us long before we begin cruising. And today we tend to look at sexuality as an either/or situation. One is or one isn't.

Gore Vidal, who has often recounted a night spent with Jack Kerouac, the aggro, hetero heartthrob of every boho broad of his time, says there's no such thing as heterosexuals or homosexuals, only heterosexual or homosexual behavior. I think that just this once Vidal is wrong—virtually all of us lean one way or another—but he has a point. There are homosexuals and heterosexuals, but there are also bisexuals and just plain sexuals. Sexuality isn't "either/or" but a spectrum, although it has some major wavelengths on it. In reading the classics one encounters many characters who manage to work up quite an enthusiasm for both females and males. And since among these apparent bisexuals are many heroes and emperors, we can assume that this was by inclination and choice, not peer pressure.

Our culture tends toward sexual specialization; unlike in ancient Rome or Athens, we tend to go one way or the other: straight or gay. And when someone begins adulthood exploring the alternatives, they tend to settle down to one sex or the other eventually. It seems a shame, in a way, to limit oneself, but our Judeo-Christian modes are designed to accommodate straight and gay as more formal, explainable, and serious than a comparatively whimsical bisexuality.

Obviously, whatever our orientation, it's usually in our best interest to discover and recognize it as soon as possible, otherwise we may be frustrated, feel that we're missing out, and have a lot of explaining to do later. And although there is certainly a long way to go toward full acceptance and equality for gay people, the world has changed enormously in my lifetime.

In my youth the comic books all had ads in them warning us that if we went to the beach and failed to display adequate musculature, we were in danger of bullies kicking sand in our faces, much to the amusement of the females that we had previously been charming with our wit. For this reason we were advised to begin lifting weights immediately. As an adult I realized that the only people likely to kick sand in my face at the beach were small children, but it was too late. The imperative to be macho was implanted.

When I encountered Manhattan's gay world I found that being a sissy was not generally in favor. Campy, queeny behavior was still around, but it had an almost old-world quality. Most gay men now favored the butch stance, and if you strolled down to the end of Christopher Street on a weekend you'd see hundreds, if not thousands of men out for a stroll wearing black leather motorcycle jackets, blue jeans, boots, flannel shirts under hooded sweatshirts, and even cowboy gear. (They weren't dubbed The Village People for nothing.) Hypermasculinity was the mode and at clubs like the Eagle's Nest and the Spike, a leather and western dress code was strictly enforced. John Waters and I were once turned away at the door of the Anvil. We were both wearing jackets and ties and the doorman said, "Gentlemen, this is a gay bar." John was delighted to have failed muster.

There were still drag queens then and they didn't DJ. I was friends with Candy Darling, Jackie Curtis, Holly Woodlawn, and that spectacle of transgender, Divine. I personally had the honor of introducing Candy to Divine at Max's Kansas City one night, and it was like the meeting of two great ladies of Hollywood, say Garbo meeting Dietrich, with each vying to see who could express the most adoration and respect for the other. The only transvestites you'd see were in the clubs or on the streets. They were entertainers or whores. And the sissy male was definitely low man on our countercultural totem pole. Gays wanted to be a man's man or a full-on girl. The sissy, widely admired at various times in history, most recently as the extravagant Wildean aesthete, had become problematic to the point of extinction.

The sissy has always been about protracted, feminine boyishness, and the cult of the sissy touched on the Greek idea of man-boy relationships. The sissy or unmanly man was called *urning* by the Uranian cult of the nineteenth century. In 1864 Karl Heinrich Ulrichs published revolutionary theories of sexual orientation, developing a complex system of sexuality accounting for the various types of behavior and attractions, such as *uranodioning* (bisexual male), *mannlinge* (rough-trade gay), *manuring* (feminine straight male), *zwischen-urning* (pederast), *virilisierte mannlinge* (closeted gay), and *uraniaster* (situational homosexual, e.g. a prisoner).

Perhaps it was simply the culture of macho, forged in Hollywood and transmitted through mass media, that did the sissy in. Ironically many of the tough guys of the Hollywood films that forged the macho persona have been retroactively outed—Rock Hudson, Randolph Scott, Tyrone Power, Gary Cooper, and Spencer Tracy. Cultural attitudes made the delicate male an object of contempt. When he appeared in dramaturgy at all it was a figure of contemptuous fun or as a villain—from Clifton Webb as Waldo Lydecker in *Laura* to Peter Lorre and Elisha Cook Jr., respectively, as Joel Cairo and Wilmer the "gunsel" in the *Maltese Falcon* to Jonathan Harris as Dr. Smith, the cowardly scientist of *Lost in Space*.

By the enlightened twentieth century, "girlie man" was the phrase chosen by California governor Arnold Schwarzenegger, who spent most of his life making a living wearing a posing strap, to insult opponents of George H. W. Bush in the 1988 election. Presumably, he meant that the legislature was a bunch of *urnings*.

One of the unintended consequences of gay liberation was that acceptance seems to have toned down "la différence" to the point that it has almost disappeared. Everybody dresses regular and talks regular. It's all so regular. I think the cultural melding of the gay and straight is inevitable, and never will we see the polarization of gender mutants that we once had. The extremes seem doomed. But maybe along with straighter gays will come gayer straights. The thing to remember about culture is that anything is possible. Hetero men will please their women by any means necessary. And so the grandness and over-the-topness that seems doomed may return among men of all preferences.

I like the swagger Johnny Depp brought to his portrayals of Lord Rochester in *The Libertine* and Captain Jack Sparrow in *Pirates of the Caribbean*. We can't forget the lessons of glitter. David Bowie, Marc Bolan, and Mick Jagger demonstrated that the guys who are in touch with their feminine side have an edge in touching the feminine insides. Sometimes the guys with girlfriends make the best girly men. Maybe it's because heteros have nothing to lose by championing the louche, faggy posture. I say to my disjunctive brothers (i.e., according to Ulrichs, those "with tender feelings for men but passionate feelings for women") that if we succeed, maybe we'll get to wear lots of velvet, mince around overdecorated homes, and have a new "Restoration" all our own.

Fashion is certainly doing its part. Page through men's fashion magazines and you'll see bold inversion displayed even in the advertising: wimps, sissies, nancy boys, and mincing weenies. They're here, they're queer, and they're in fashion. Look what they're selling to men.

There's the flaming-red-haired Lanvin boy with the come-hither eyeliner and lipsticked pout; the CK boys who look as if every hair but those on their scalps and brows has been waxed away; the limp-wristed Daks dweeb who's all brow and temples; the Dior boys with toothpick arms, no body hair, and no trace of beard; and the Burberry boys who stand there, puzzled, with Kate Moss (maybe their babysitter?); and the Jil Sander guy, awkwardly slumped in a corner, who reminds me of the kid I used to strong-arm to help me out in physics lab. I love the Jil Sander clothes. I have that crewneck sweater myself. But I must say, the emotion that the young man projects is pathos. He evokes pity, sympathy, and compassion. I want to buy that sweater just to cheer him up. It's the absolute inverse of everything taught in Marketing 101. Nike says "Just Do It." Jil Sander says nothing but suggests, "Please, don't hurt me." Ah, fashion certainly takes interesting positions. They come from what former President Bush calls "the gut," and certainly not from market research. And that's what's great about fashion. The gut.

My gut tells me that the world is changing. Pee-wee Herman was a prophet. Sasha Baron Cohen's Bruno is coming. The world is overpopulated. The world's imperial power flails away in military disasters. Sports records fall to steroid mutants on amphetamines and HGH. Right-wing pundit Ann Coulter gets cheered for calling Democratic presidential candidate John Edwards a faggot. Clearly we are in the midst of a gender identity crisis. It's time to be a man. But be a man in splendor and magnificence and eloquence—not in brute silence.

What is the answer to the neoconservatives, the Islamic fundamentalists, twelve-step earnestness, and Scientology? Maybe it's mass cultural extravagance. Bring on the sissies, the fops, and high fashion. Fashion is the one thing I can imagine taking young men's minds off institutional religion, which to me is nothing but failed fagginess. We need a brave new fagginess that will blow the Pope's red shoes right out of the water and make the Taliban's heavy-handed mascara run from weeping. Straight men need to find their flamboyance. We need gay men to be gayer too. We need straight men to take up the kilt and swish with abandon. Bend it like Beckham! We need a new superficiality that can challenge the insane illusions that pass for reality in the media.

Since the world's religions have spent the last millennium disgracing themselves, what have we left to believe in but fashion? It is more faith-based than anything else I can think of, and yet it doesn't contradict science. And it is completely harmless. Its uselessness is positively Buddhist in its militant inaction. As the world goes to hell I can only think of Peter Pan and the dying Tinkerbell and chant: "I do believe in fairies. I do believe in fairies." It's going to take their kind of magic to get us out of this macho-made mess.

The military still says "Don't ask, don't tell." Shame on them! I say, "Ask everyone! Spill the beans!" Do you like girls? Marvelous! Do you like boys? Fabulous! We don't need undercover lovers or wolves dressed in priests' clothing; we need proud shamans who can do the voodoo they do so well. Yes, it was a shame that the Army fired all those Arabic-speaking translators because they came out of the closet. But if the intelligence agencies were really intelligent, they'd bombard our medieval opponents, such as the Taliban, with Queen records and Galliano fashions. Maybe they wouldn't hate women so much if they could be one on the weekend. Come out, come out, wherever you are!

It's the twenty-first century, gentlemen, and roles are changing. And at my house everybody wears the pants and brings home the bacon. I'm just a modern guy. Of course I've had it in the ear before. I've got a lust for life. So what can I say? I can box out and I can gift wrap. I play from the blue tees but I make the risotto in my house. The divisions of labor are a-changing. I am not what my ancestors had in mind: I don't plow or wear a sword, but on the reproductive front I am getting the job done. I am evolution. I am the new man. Hear me roar: We're here, we're sometimes mistaken for queer—get used to it.

1   I just learned Gaydar really exists. It's a phone app called Grindr.

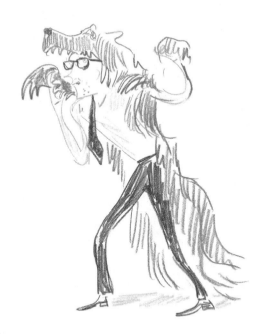

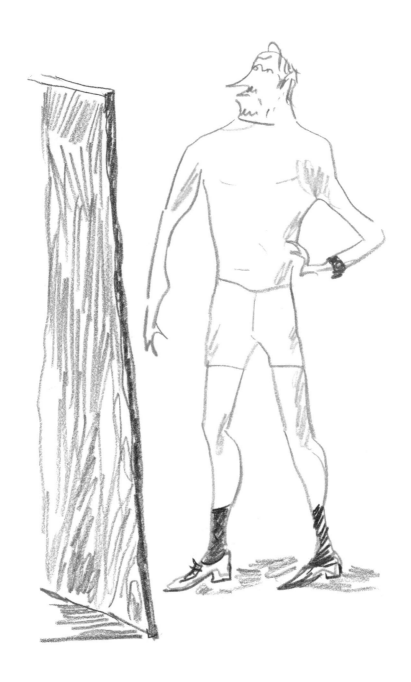

HOW TO NOT LOOK STUPID

Most men's education in dressing went something like this: "Here, put this on."

As boys, we are dressed in protective coverings and asked to try to keep them clean. We are given overalls for coverage, sneakers for traction, and T-shirts that amuse our mothers with sayings we don't understand. The fanciful among us, not content with "happy face" T-shirts and denim, may discover more expressive clothes through our peers or by observing the world's entertainment and begin to form our own ideas of style based on these.

Recalling my own childhood, I realize that much of my time was spent in costume—army combat fatigues, cow-punching gear (including boots, chaps, vest, and scaled-down ten-gallon hat), flight suits, baseball jerseys, and so on. I see this pattern repeated by my ten-year-old son, who often greets visitors in SWAT team getup or as Darth Vader, complete with the museum-quality light saber. Luckily, his size defuses what could be a scary occasion. Girls, however, tend to be trained from an early age to be civilians and to develop an appropriate sense of occasion. Girls are often educated in a style of dress by their mothers, while boys are left to pick up a sense of role from the media and fall into a general cluelessness that is passed down from generation to generation.

Looking good, or actually looking right, is not high on the cultural curriculum of the American male, and learning to present himself in public is not easy. At every turn, it seems, he will be encouraged to look stupid. If he shows originality or style, he may be mocked by his peers. If he shows up dressed inappropriately for an occasion, it is unlikely anyone will set him straight.

The Jews have the right idea with the bar mitzvah. Every culture should be a tribal ritual or tradition informing the boy that he has become a man and that he'd better get with the program. He should probably, at that point, publicly change from shorts to trousers, appearing to applause in a suit and tie and burning his baseball cap. Unfortunately we have no common coming-of-age ceremony. Girls have their sweet sixteen while boys are told they should get a job at Starbucks, and so it seems that many men, even those gray with age, have no idea that they are not boys anymore.

In many quarters males are trained (often by default) to seek comfort in their clothing as an ideal. Meanwhile, it is suggested that other motivations in dressing are suspect. It's a scene reenacted endlessly in popular entertainment and situation comedy—the wife's attempts to throw out her husband's moth-eaten jacket and his pathetic protests. Males are creatures of habit and so they often settle on a sort of uniform that gets them through the day. They become attached to a certain item, a jacket or sweatshirt as a fetish, a Linus security blanket that makes them feel safe and serves as a talisman against struggle and decision.

Historically, boys have gotten increasingly dressed up as they moved toward manhood, sometimes in a school uniform with the old-school tie, sometimes observing a school or church dress code, like white shirt and tie, designed to prepare them for the world of business. Sometimes they resisted putting on the shirt, tie, and jacket, as it represented duty and responsibility, and so it was fought against—particularly the necktie—as restrictive or uncomfortable, but still they knew that donning the proper clothes was inevitable.

Now the casualization of dress has made men question previously unassailable standards. It has become increasingly possible for men to dress like boys or adolescents for life. We see these fellows around us every day. They are the chaps in comfy running shoes, worn jeans, tracksuits, sweats, T-shirts, and caps advertising the sports teams to which they hold allegiance. These men are dressed not for success but for existence. For them, clothing's function is to prevent nudity and therefore embarrassment and to ensure that they blend in and not appear discernibly different from their buddies. They dress for homely invisibility.

I often see young men on dates, dressed in T-shirts, jeans, and sneakers, accompanying well-groomed, prettily clad girls in dresses and high heels, and it looks like they are going to entirely different places. I somehow hope that the fellow is a chauffeur or even a bodyguard, but I know better and I think, Where did our culture go off the rails?

Even in business one sees this phenomenon of mass unconsciousness: we see men in business suits who appear unable to actually see themselves. Their suits seem to have been made for much larger bodies. Perhaps, you think, this fellow plans to gain a hundred pounds, or is he that guy who lost a hundred pounds eating at Subway? Trousers bunch up around their shoes, jacket cuffs hang to the knuckles. These are company men; they are executives, even. But when you look closer at a group of suits, you see that not all are alike. Some in the pack seem to wear suits that adhere more reasonably to their bodies, and we make a mental note that these are the young alphas, the future chiefs of that corporate tribe, because men without vanity, with no ability to perceive themselves in the mirror, are fated to be drones.

The manifestation of style is something a man has to learn for himself. Style can be taught, but some students are too damaged to be capable of absorbing the lessons. Women tend to have a keener sense of men's style than men do, since part of their role is responding to it in their quest for the alpha male, but their advice is often disregarded because they are female. Many men consider attention to one's person a feminine trait, not only an interest in clothing but even in matters of grooming such as removing their

God-given body hair. Some men, however, perhaps the boys who did get some attentive mothering, are all too happy to let the wife pick out all their clothes. They may look better, but at what cost?

Style is the visible manifestation of personality. According to psychology a personality is constructed by identification—a process in which a subject assimilates attributes of another and is transformed, wholly or partially, after the model the other provides.

So style generally begins in identifying with and mimicking an admired person, whether the role model is within one's circle or a celebrity. A man may aspire to the style of a mentor or he may pick a model from the pantheon of publicity—an actor, a musician, a politician, an athlete, or an entrepreneur that he feels he can relate to and with whom he feels a psychological kinship. Walking the streets of a major city it's easy to catalog the primary molds in which men cast themselves.

Today we see packs of young men cavorting in mimesis of the characters of the HBO show *Entourage*. There's the chubby one in the Yankees cap, Turtle; the affably overconfident, muscular yob, Drama; the cocky, preppy, E; the chick magnet, Vince. A similar phenomenon gripped society some years back when single adult women began drinking and talking dirty in packs, acting out roles cut whole cloth (leopard-skin spandex) from *Sex and the City*.

Personality cloning from the media is no accident. Television's precise function seems to be organizing society into a hive of sorts, creating informal but effective flowcharts of personality. The old class system as defined by the Industrial Revolution is no longer operative. Today's information society requires types more diverse and complex than the Bob Cratchits, Ebenezer Scrooges, Howard Roarks, and Longfellow Deedses who informed twentieth-century society.

Even society's fringes are peopled by media archetypes. The Village People were one such cocktail of hypermasculine tropes, and decades later we still see overcompensatory style choices. In an increasingly conformist society we see more and more samplings from the repertoire of the rebel—the Brando biker, the Jack Sparrow pirate-dandy, the beatnik of fifty years ago, the hippie of forty years ago, and the punk rocker of thirty years ago. History may have passed them by, but they still hang out on the corner.

Our identification with celebrities is inevitable and sometimes useful. Even celebrities do it. Could there have been a George Clooney without a Cary Grant? A Brad Pitt without a Gary Cooper? Information is transmitted by acting it out, and we are the electrons and megabytes in the big machine. But to achieve success in life and work, it is important that one doesn't look stupid, like an imitation. Like a good actor plays a written role, we refine it until it is ours.

Avoiding looking stupid and clichéd is not as easy as one would think, because it is far easier to fall back on effective clichés than to compose something original. Clichés are powerful. They move the masses. Donald Trump is a success because he has perfected himself as a cliché. Anyone who has created a talking doll that repeats seventeen of his oft-repeated sayings at the pull of a string has himself become that doll. "Think big and live large...stay focused...I should fire myself just for having you around."

Donald Trump is a great success because he has become a hieroglyph of wealth in the media vernacular. (In fact he redefined wealth, turning an ability to incur vast debt into a perception of vast wealth.) Trump has gone viral. He has become contagious. His image DNA is loose in the system. He is reproducing an army of clones. Would we have a Rod Blagojevich if there were no Donald Trump?

So as we negotiate this galaxy of reality shows that is contemporary culture, we cannot avoid role models. There are only so many prototypes. Supposedly there are thirty-six archetypal dramatic situations. There are eighty-five possible ways to knot a necktie. There are forty-six chromosomes in the human genome. We all begin as types. Some of us, like the foxy Nexus-6 replicants of *Blade Runner,* may even develop emotions and believe our memories are not implants. We begin as types but if we do our job as men, we end up prototypes. Pass it on.

The best role models are complex and distant. George Clooney is not a bad choice for a role model, but a character he plays, Michael Clayton, is probably a better choice because he is more complex, indefinable, and abstract. Like acting, life is a quest for good scripts. If personality is, in a sense, a container, then our job is to fill it with the most exquisite and beautiful content. We must balance our sense-acquired knowledge of the world with the lore of culture, passed down through art and literature. And then, when we have gathered the best we can find, it's time to improvise.

In the liner notes to Miles Davis's *Kind of Blue*, Bill Evans wrote:

> "…conviction that direct deed is the most meaningful reflection, I believe, has prompted the evolution of the extremely severe and unique disciplines of the jazz or improvising musician."

Who looks stupid? The wallflower who just sits there, afraid of action, or the guy who's good to go, even if sometimes half-cocked? The man of action might make a mistake, but sometimes it's better to do it wrong than to do nothing at all. Trial and error is how we earn our chops. And if the man of action screws up, it's harder to notice because his velocity makes him a little blurry. That's OK. Style is a work in progress. "By the time they catch us," said Ishmael Reed, "we're not there."

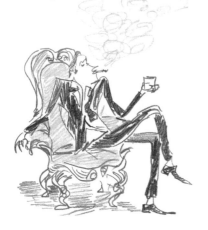

NOTES ON THE DANDY

"Fastidious, unbelievables, beaux, lions, or dandies: whichever label these men claim for themselves, one and all stem from the same origin, all share the same characteristic of opposition and revolt; all are representatives of what is best in human pride, of that need, which is too rare in the modern generation, to combat and destroy triviality."

—Charles Baudelaire, "The Dandy," from *The Painter of Modern Life*

What do you call guys like us? Men who pay attention to how we look. Men who like clothes and put some thought into them. Who care about being well groomed and living in a beautiful place. Who think that art isn't just something that goes onto a canvas or up and down in value, but something that informs the way we live.

Being called a man-about-town is OK, but we want to look good in the country too. "Clotheshorse" puts too much emphasis on the clothes and not enough on the man. We're not centaurs and a suit ain't a saddle. "Fashion plate"? No, style isn't fashion, and I refuse to think of myself as a plate or any other sort of container. "Fop"? Fightin' words, pally. Would you say that to Sinatra? "Mondain" or "boulevardier" has a certain ring-a-ding-ding, but those tags won't play in Chicago. "Natty" is old school, but it's a little skeezy. If you're going to be natty you've got to be dreaded as well. I've been called "flaneur" a couple of times lately in blogs, and I like that, but I think I work too hard for it to be a perfect fit.

"Metrosexual"? That was the last pop construct: the man who likes women but who has the same sort of aesthetic orientation as men who like men. The metrosexual has been defined many ways, but basically it comes down to being a participant in fashion, which usually means a victim. I'd prefer fashion combatant, meaning that whatever style I manifest is in the arena and I'm in it to win it.

Good old "dandy," however, is something I can live with. "Dandy" is a good word, even if it's often misunderstood. Not only does it state a case for pride and creative elegance, but it also provides a historical context that is meaningful, even inspiring. Imagine that the act of putting your clothes on in the morning can be a philosophical, political, or even revolutionary act. What shakes up the establishment? Nothing gets the goat of an old fogy more than a splendid dandy in full strut, exhibiting his flamboyant individuality like a male peacock in the throes of rampant display. I don't recall my parents' generation being scared by Abbie Hoffman, Jerry Rubin, and the other self-proclaimed revolutionaries dedicated to the destruction of the capitalist war machine, but I do remember parents being up in arms when the Rolling Stones appeared on *The Ed Sullivan Show*. A classmate's dad broke all of his son's Stones albums. I don't know if it was Mick Jagger's exaggerated mincing or Brian Jones wearing what looked like a Lilly Daché lady's hat that did it, but the old man was clearly threatened by a style that made him feel obsolete.

The dread that man felt looking at his son's idols was similar to what he might have felt looking at a pimp dressed in a green velvet suit and a big Stetson hat, driving a custom Caddy with a sunroof top and a diamond in the back. What sends emasculatory chills through the hearts of the salary-men we call "suits" are the cool cats unashamed to be dandies. Men who are proud of themselves, of their faces and bodies and their tastes; men who stand out from the pack so diligently playing follow-the-leader.

Let's dismiss any shred of an idea that a dandy is a fop, a coxcomb, a poseur, or a pretender. Let me quote the learned Lord Whimsy on the subject, from his book *The Affected Provincial's Companion*:

"Contrary to conventional wisdom, the dandy is not merely a preening vacant popinjay; for in truth, he is a preening thoughtful popinjay. Dandyism pertains to more than the wearing of clothes: it is a way of being, a philosophy. The dandy's attire is but an outer expression of his inner refinement—the delicate glass that holds a finely crafted wine."

A dandy isn't faking it. A dandy may begin as a poseur, but gradually the pose takes hold and gives him strength, and though he may have begun as a phony, by affecting a grand posture, the power of the posture reforms him and he becomes a real phony. Although a dandy can be effete, he is just as likely to be tough as nails. Sugar Ray Leonard, Smokin' Joe Frazier, and Oscar de la Hoya are all dandies, as was Cassius Clay/Muhammad Ali at the height of his prowess, not to mention the great heavyweight Jack Johnson, and the welterweight Frank Sinatra.

A dandy is not a fop, a metrosexual or, inherently, a sissy; however, a sissy, through hard work and commitment, may attain the state of dandyism if he doesn't settle for foppery. Dandies can be dangerous and a dandy might fight over a derogatory comment on his attire, should a witty riposte prove insufficient punishment. He will not fly into a senseless rage, though, but a sensible rage, and will perhaps prevail upon a bystander to hold his jacket while he kicks a poorly furnished ass. Dandies have been known to join an army or a navy in part because of their admiration for the uniform. (That's why the great Beau Brummell joined the Tenth Hussars—it was the best-dressed regiment in the British Army.) Is not every U.S. Marine a dandy in a way? Many dandies have led armies and fleets, and as generals or admirals they have the prerogative to design their own uniforms, as did such dandies as Generals Eisenhower, Patton, and MacArthur.

Dandies are a certain breed of men. They notice what others are wearing and they have an opinion about it. But that's a small part of the story. Dandies tend to have opinions about everything. Dandies know art, architecture, food and drink, literature and dance, maybe even sports. You might think you know who the dandies are and what they stand for, but perhaps you don't. Dandies have secrets. Maybe dandydom is a sort of secret society, a fraternity that recognizes its membership not by secret words or signs but by overtly inimitable design.

Every dandy begins with one thing: pride. The dandy loves himself, and, by extension, mankind and the world. But the dandy's pride is not vanity. The true dandy thinks he has good reason to love himself. The fop also seems to love himself, but in fact it is his own reflection that the fop loves. Dandyism is not narcissism—it is applied art. It applies everything we have learned about aesthetics and from philosophy to our persons and to our environments. Dandyism is a glorification of oneself for reasons that may, ultimately, be selfless. It is a philosophy of the transcendent self.

Charles Baudelaire wrote:

"Contrary to what a lot of thoughtless people seem to believe, dandyism is not even an excessive delight in clothes and material elegance. For the perfect dandy, these things are no more than the symbol of the aristocratic superiority of his mind."

The dandy is not a disciple of Freud or, in all likelihood, the Buddha. To the dandy, the ego, the I, is something to nourish, not something to lose. The dandy may be quite spiritual in outlook, considering his body a temple and its raiment a glorification of the divine form. Dandyism approaches a sort of profane religiosity. The dandy is not a puritan. He doesn't generally talk to God, although he may well try to channel him in order to emulate and propagate the grandeur attributed to the deity. Except for clerics, who are often dandies (particularly those of the Roman persuasion), the dandy is not particularly concerned with the judgment of God except as interpreted by himself. The dandy doesn't second-guess. He prefers knowledge to belief. If he is a believer at all, he is probably a deist or a pagan, a polytheist who finds the division of divine labor more entertaining and picturesque than authoritarian monotheism. Above all the dandy is a philosopher who believes in reason and the evidence of his own senses, in his own taste and, to some extent, the approbation of his respected peers.

This is, however, a rough time for philosophy. At a 2007 Republican presidential debate, three of ten candidates raised their hands when asked, "Who does not believe in evolution?" A 2006 Pew Research survey found that 40 percent of American Christians believe Jesus will return by 2050. It seems more and more that America has reached a cultural crisis, with the deity about to write some big blank checks that the believers can't wait to cash. We seem to be on the verge of discovering what democracy means in an ignorant society. The next decade could make the execution of Socrates by the Athenian democracy seem like chump change.

Civilized people will have to abandon their casual, laissez-faire stance, at least temporarily, in order to retake control of the world from religious pretenders supposedly in the confidence of an activist God. They've got them in Tehran and we've got them in Washington and believers in imaginary realms shouldn't be running a planet. Philosophy is needed now more than ever, but these are such unphilosophical times that perhaps it must be sold as something else, like entertainment or fashion or, best of all, style, that greatest surviving domain of individuality.

A dandy can't just focus on style and ignore the big picture. It is fine for him to be familiar with Epicurious.com, but he should also know Epicurus (341–270 BCE), whose materialism became known as Epicureanism. Epicurus fought well against the prevailing superstitions of his day, which are pretty much the same as those of our day, such as divine intervention. He demonstrated that pain was bad and pleasure was good and that it's important to watch your back. Baudelaire also linked dandyism to the Greek philosophical school of Stoicism (suppressed by the Christian emperor Justinian in 529). Stoicism still exists today, wherever it is said "living well is the best revenge."

The original dandy was a flower in the lapel of Enlightenment, but that sort has vanished. As Baudelaire wrote:

"But alas! The rising tide of democracy, which spreads everywhere and reduces everything to the same level, is daily carrying away these last champions of human pride, and submerging, in the waters of oblivion, the last traces of these remarkable myrmidons."

The dandy exists today, but he is often a solitary or marginalized figure. What once empowered the dandy was solidarity with his fellows. Joined together, dandies will not only be powerful, they will have a great deal of fun amazing the world. If the Republican Right can re-brand themselves as the Tea Party, surely there is room for an Arty Party consisting of dandies, male and female, to throw a political party that will stand up for ideas rather than slogans.

Philosophically, the dandy lives in the present. Like Epicurus, he believes that pleasure and pain are the indicators of good and evil and that the hereafter is not only irrelevant, but it is a fraud foisted upon us by the jealous. And because dandies do tend to live in the present moment, I believe they will find themselves at an advantage over those who are always looking aloft for a Second Coming. But even if Jesus does return in the near future, we will be sure that he is properly dressed, fed, and entertained, and we will be sure to inform him of all the misdeeds of those in the habit of speaking and acting on his behalf.

The founding dandy, Beau Brummell, was the first celebrity. In a way he was a very modern celebrity because he was not famous so much for doing something as being something. Anne Hollander wrote in *Sex and Suits:*

"In the new urban Dandy mode, a man's heroism consists only in being himself; Brummell proved that the essential superior being was no longer a hereditary nobleman. His excellence was entirely personal, unsupported by armorial bearings, ancestral halls, vast lands or even a fixed address… His garments had to be perfect only in their own sartorial integrity, that is in form alone, unburdened by any surface indices of the worth attached to rank."

Before Brummell, men wore ostentatious fashion with lots of gold braid, frill, and filigree. Brummell's clothes were monochromatic, black, gray, navy, or buff, and without decoration. He introduced the ultimately practical garment: trousers. He wore no cosmetics and no perfumes and was notoriously obsessed with clean linen, washed and dried in the country. Brummell's revolution was about modernity, simplicity, practicality, cleanliness, fitness of body, and clothes that fit. He said—somewhat tongue in cheek but making his point—that if you were noticed on the street you had failed. Richard Faulk wrote that Brummell believed "the thorough gentleman is exceptional only in the extraordinary perfection of his ordinariness."

In his enlightening 1951 study *Clothes*, James Laver wrote:

"...the greatest dandy of all was, of course, Beau Brummell, and it was he who was the protagonist, if not the originator of the new doctrine of gentility, the sociological innovation which is behind dandyism. We shall never understand Gentility unless we realize that it was, in one of its aspects, a conspiracy against the aristocracy. Brummell himself was a parvenu, yet he made himself the acknowledged *arbiter elegantiarum*, the veritable tyrant of the mode. The Prince Regent himself is said to have burst into tears when Brummell told him his breeches did not fit."

Beau Brummell created a modern fashion, but he wasn't thinking of creating a fashion. He was manifesting his own style, first for himself and then for the general enlightenment of society, and that style drew followers. Fashion is only useful if it serves the individual, giving him a context in which he can distinguish himself. Otherwise fashion is like religion, an opiate for the masses. We're living in a time of revolution. The American political system no longer resembles the one we grew up in. A massive redistribution of wealth has occurred that dwarfs that of the robber barons and the gilded age. The media, meanwhile, focuses on a small cast of "controversial" celebrities and promotes a universal devotion to fashion and sex gossip.

Today we need style, more than ever, to shake society out of its luxury coma. Perhaps things are less obvious for us in America, but the kids in Tehran know that fashion is politics, and the girl in her Hermès scarf or the boy who looks too much like Brad Pitt is risking arrest. They are still trying to make the twentieth century happen in their society. But we've to get the twenty-first going. There was a time not so long ago when long hair could get your car stopped and bell-bottoms could land you in a lineup. That was true Dandyism, revolutionary sex appeal for a New Age. It was the revolution of the rockers and the mods, the hippies and the Black Panthers with their black leather, big Afros, and berets.

There's always a status quo, and there is always an avant-garde, a cadre of the cleverly turned out that understands the meaning behind appearance and its social and political impact. I remember well when spontaneously formed armies of freaks in elaborate and outlandish personal costume brought down a president and stopped a war. There are lines in the sand, and lines on suit makers' patterns. Sometimes you need to step over them all. Remember the words of George Clinton: "If you've got funk, you've got style."

It may seem like we've become a nation of sheep, but that can only mean that the hour of the wolf is near. It's time to put on the dog and get ready for Riding Hood. Calling all rakehells and bohos, all dandies and beaux, all dreadlocks and zoot suits, all hipsters and swanks, all mods and rockers. Conformity has given us nothing but war, boredom, misery, and bad television. We must dress as only we can. We must dress up and over-the-top to show the world that we aren't huddled masses but individual characters, ready to do our own thing flamboyantly at the drop of a beret. Together we'll change the world, one stitch at a time.

ON SUITS

A man must wear a suit. He must not be a suit. The suit works for you, pally, you don't work for it. You paid the cost, so be the boss. Wear it. Don't let it wear you.

Some men wear a suit only when they wed and when they're dead. Some men wear a suit only when they are tried and when they're laid out. But the suit is not just for those occasions when your name appears in the papers. Many men put on the suit on Sunday-to-go-to-meeting; for some it's the uniform, Monday through Friday, the management uniform, the frame for the white collar and tie. For some it is simply what a gentleman wears in default mode. For others it's dressing up, for one reason or another. It is as good as it gets; the suit is eminently suitable.

The modern suit was originally called a lounge suit, and it was intended not for the professional on duty but for the gentleman off duty. It was an informal dress-up ensemble for entertaining at home or traveling. The frock coat and striped pants with wing collar was still the working ensemble of the man-about-town. But after the Great War, as the twenties began to roar, the Jazz Age required a more limber mode for doing the Black Bottom, the Charleston, and the Lindy Hop, and for fleeing from speakeasies during police raids. The frock coat and striped trousers persisted for a while but began to look aged and stuffy, and finally the frock coat was worn only by clerks and the hired help. By the late twenties the lounge suit was the universal public look of the urbane male. He wore it to work and he could wear it out for the evening too, unless he had time to go home and dress for dinner in his tuxedo, which was basically a deluxe lounge suit.

Tailless, trim, and made of one fabric, top and bottom, the suit was a perfect costume for the rise of modernism. Sleek rather than stiff, trimmed of tails that might get caught in the cogs of the machine age, the suit was ready for work and play, and with plenty of pockets it was ready for upward mobility and management of the corporations that would rule the world.

What distinguished one suit from another was mainly its color.

Black: for funerals and the clergy.

Dark gray: suitable for all occasions.

Light gray: normal business and social wear.

Navy blue: suitable for most occasions; not as dressy as dark gray.

Olive green: for the stylish brave; for the warrior of the creative department and the rootless traveling salesman.

There are businesses and there are businesses. Wall Street and banking have always tended toward the conservative suit, and the man in the gray flannel suit had more than one in the closet. Serious firms favored a sober, conservative look and for the most part suits other than dark gray and navy were "simply not done." Through most of the twentieth century, proper gents would not have worn a brown or green suit to the office. It would have been considered too "racetrack" or too country, although who wears a suit to the track or the farm these days, I can't imagine. Ironically the brown suit was redeemed by that idol of conservatives, Ronald Reagan. There are still firms where brown is not worn, or plaids, but the codes have eroded and are upheld mostly by frivolous fussbudgets and cloutless curmudgeons.

In the late twenties stripes appeared, borrowed from tennis apparel, and they caught on with stylish men everywhere, though in conservative firms a man had to earn his stripes. Glen plaids, herringbones, and textured fabrics caught on with fashionable men about town, and peaked lapels and double-breasted jackets gave the urbane gent many options.

Pinstripes or chalk stripes have been considered a sharp business look for so long that the association with the gangster movies that helped popularize them has been forgotten. Pinstripes are more formal than chalk stripes, which are bold and can be slightly wise-guy looking, depending on who's wearing them. I wouldn't wear chalk stripes to a trial if I were a litigant or defendant, although they could work on counsel. I would never wear chalk stripes to a funeral unless I was celebrating. The usual suit stripe is in fairly high contrast, like white or off-white on navy or gray, or navy on white or off-white. In recent years we have been seeing more colored stripes, such as red or green on navy or gray. These contrasts are obviously less dressy than the traditional white stripe. We have even seen Hollywoodish tailors turn their clients' names or initials into stripes of fine print, a practice that verges on unspeakable.

Plaids have been urbane business-wear for many decades and are acceptable in most any circle. The more creative your business, the bolder your plaid can be. If you are a CEO, you can wear glen plaid on an average workday. If you are an editor at *Vogue*, you can have a full tartan run up into a suit. Very plaid suits, bold checks, and windowpanes, like tweeds, fall into the realm of the sporty or country suit, but in this casual era the lines have blurred. Once tweeds were considered country wear, but who wears suits in the country anymore, even when we are shooting at things or exercising our quadrupeds? These traditional favorites seem to still thrive on campus and might take the train into the city on cold days when the calendar is easy.

Suitings, the fabrics used to make suits, have changed considerably over the last half century as climate control has eliminated much of the real need for insulating menswear. Offices and cars are the same temperature year-round, and central heating has even conquered London. Thus suit fabrics have lightened up and winter weights practically disappeared. Once wool that weighed sixteen ounces a yard was common in northern climes. Now we see men wearing eight-ounce wool year-round. Caution, please. There is no such thing as a suit for all seasons.

White or cream is perfect for a summer suit. It was almost extinct for years, as we went through a laid-back, blend-in period, but now it's back in its full brilliance. And light suits in a wide variety of shades pop out like flowers in June. A decade or so ago seersucker was kept alive by the bold few (including bold conservatives) and was generally found with blue, gray, or brown stripes only. Today we find seersuckers with pink, orange, red, or green stripes.

Tan suits are really appropriate only for fair weather, although you'd never know that by looking at NBA benches. We see coaches and injured players wearing tan suits all winter. Maybe this is because men with brown complexions look so good in tan and light brown suits. The rule? If you are good-looking enough, you can break the rules.

It's a fact that men of black and brown complexion can pull off suits that pinker cats can't. I love the wild-colored suits that British custom tailor Ozwald Boateng makes and wears, but I have to admit I just can't wear an orange suit. But there are white men who can. The trademark of the natty Knight Landesman, the publisher of *Artforum,* is wearing bright-colored suits in any season, which makes it easy to find him at any art fair. He's the guy in the fire-engine-red or canary-yellow suit. In the art world, there is no wrong-colored suit.

Pockets

Once, according to tailor/historian Alan Flusser, who knows such things, all pockets were flapless. Then that sartorial maverick, Edward, Prince of Wales (later, briefly, Edward VIII of England, and eventually the Duke of Windsor), created a vogue for the flap. Flapped pockets are more casual, hence their absence from tuxedos and dinner jackets. Better flap-pocket suit jackets feature a double besom, a welted edge above and below the pocket slit that enables the flap to be worn inside invisibly. If that's the case with your jacket, it's your choice. (Although if you affect a ticket pocket you're stuck with flaps.) But with a bulky tweed sport jacket, I doubt the flaps will go quietly.

The Ready-made Suit

Once upon a time, if you wanted a suit, you went to a tailor and he made one up for you. Then in the 1840s the automatic sewing machine was invented and ready-made suits hit the market. Brooks Brothers introduced the concept in 1845, and it was an enormous success. Before long, manufacturers were ready-making suits of a quality that was competitive with the hand-tailored genuine article. Companies like Hickey Freeman combined craftsmanship with technology to churn out high-quality clothing that could pass in the boardroom and at the club, and you didn't have to have a guy with a tape measure all over you and you didn't have to wait. The other benefit of a ready-to-wear suit was that it was cheaper. Not necessarily cheap, but cheaper.

Today ready-to-wear suits from fashion designers and premium menswear companies can cost as much or more than a bespoke or custom-made suit. In the store they may have decorative basting around them and lack buttons so they look unfinished, but that's all for show.

Why are these suits so expensive? Some of them are made from luxurious materials. If you're going to buy a cashmere suit, it's going to cost you. Some are made in factories where the workers are paid in pounds, euros, or dollars—not in yuan. And then some are made by designers who spend a lot of money on advertising. Let's see... Prada suit: $2,495. Lanvin tux: $2,900. Richard James off-the-peg: $1,795. Belvest: $2,895. Kiton: $4,495. All ready-made. Wow.

Bespoke tailors, like Anderson & Sheppard or my man John Pearse, who has a little shop in Soho, aren't spending pounds on advertising. The substantial prices of their garments reflect the cost of labor (and the state of the dollar.) I figure if I'm going to spend a lot of money on a suit, it might as well be exactly what I want and made to fit my body. And amortized over a decade, they're not really expensive.

But for years, I did buy off-the-rack and I did fine. My body was well within minor alteration range. So what do you look for in a ready-made suit? The basic aesthetic decision is the silhouette, or style, of the suit. Do you want a full-cut traditional American sack suit, with little or no waist suppression, or do you want a more British cut that fits closer to the body?

It's not about the name on the label but the fit. Every company that makes suits makes them for a certain man. They have a fit model. "Off-the-peg" suits are made to fit that designer's median customer. The buyer's strategy should be to find the house with the fit model closest to him in physique. Some suits are made for thinner guys, some for bigger, some for more athletic. And a brand may change its fit from year to year, depending on fashion.

In recent years we've seen an increase in drop—a term referring to the difference between the jacket size and trouser size. A size 42 with a six-inch drop would mean the trousers have a 36 waist. Some brands might offer an eight-inch drop. The most crucial element of the fit is in the shoulders. Most other areas can be adjusted, but the shoulders are the backbone of a suit.

Then consider how the suit was made. The question you want answered is, how was the jacket constructed? Is it full canvas, half canvas or fused? The traditional construction, which you'll find in bespoke clothing and most (but scarily not all) expensive clothing, is full canvas. There is a middle structural layer to which the front and back of the jacket are attached or basted, i.e., sewn loosely with hand stitching so the garment will move with you. If you wear your suits frequently, canvas construction is well worth the extra cost. It looks better, particularly when you move, and it will last much longer. The glue in fused jackets ages and sometimes reacts with dry-cleaning chemicals. The front of the jacket may even bubble, and then it's trash.

We are often told that fusing and the glues used in the process have improved, and that may be true, but generally speaking such suits are not a good investment. This matter is complicated by half-canvased jackets, which combine the techniques. Sometimes the chest is canvased while the lapels are fused. These jackets achieve a softer effect than a full-on glue job, but again there is a risk of bubbling, and you don't get a nice soft feel to the lapels. If your salesperson doesn't know how a suit is constructed, he is in the wrong business, or he's lying and should be arrested by the fashion police, who are never around when you need them.

Fashion vs. Eternity

There are more styles available now than ever before. Fashion suits are generally inspired by Hedi Slimane's very slim Dior clothes or Thom Browne's short-jacket-and-skinny-pants take on Ivy League. Do fashion suits lack longevity? Who knows? My late stepfather's early-sixties Hickey Freeman suit looks precisely in fashion today, except for the trousers, which have about three inches more rise. (Rise is the length from crotch to waistband.) The tide goes out and the tide comes in. That's fashion. But in general, men's clothing changes very slowly. A classic suit, styled like those offered by Savile Row or Ralph Lauren, could remain in style for a lifetime. My best suit is fifteen years old and nicely worn in. In *The Duke of Bedford's Book of Snobs*, John, the Duke, wrote:

"Suits must be made of excellent material, that goes without saying; but though they have to be new, yet they must look old. Or not too new at any rate. Filling the pockets of one's new suit with stones and hanging it out in the rain is one possible solution; another is to let your man—your valet—always wear your suits for the first two years."

Most of the suits that I have worn in my life, I could still wear today without embarrassment. I avoided the big lapels of the polyester seventies. My only errors, I think, were made under the influence of Italian designers in the nineties. Somehow those enormous shelflike shoulders looked fine back then, apparently, but in retrospect they're absurd. In a suit with heavily padded shoulders, Michael Jordan appeared to have a head the size of a grapefruit.

The blousy pleated pants of that era have dated badly too. I blame it all on coach Pat Riley. Whatever fashion is worn by athletes and coaches on television seems a must to avoid—high vests, high-roll three-button suits, and four- to six-button single-breasted suits. And incidentally, nothing can be done for your nineties "power suit"; any good tailor will tell you that the shoulders are inoperable.

My advice is, keep the shoulders naturalistic. I like a suit jacket almost as softly constructed as a sweater, with very little if any shoulder padding, a British-style nipped waist, and reasonable lapels. I am convinced that the lapels I wear—about three and three-fourths inches wide at the widest point, about four inches wide for double-breasted or peaked lapels—will never go out of style in my lifetime. If they do, civilization as we know it has ended.

Suits have long come in single-breasted and double-breasted styles. The double-breasted suit imitated a naval uniform jacket; it became popular in the thirties and remained so into the fifties, but in the sixties it nearly disappeared, being worn mostly by stubborn older men. No American president between Harry Truman and Bill Clinton wore a double-breasted suit, but today the double-breasted jacket is high style once again. It is not for children, and generally does not work well on small or short men, or on the portly. Young men usually prefer single-breasted suits, but a stylish and good-figured fellow of any age can pull off double-breasted. Where do you draw the line? Bill Clinton, at his peak weight, was pushing the double-breasted envelope.

Even when the double-breasted suit was out with the suit-wearing masses, it retained a foothold in fashion. The radical tailors who made "Mod" and "Carnaby Street" household terms liked to play with that style, along with the Nehru and other occult cuts, and they revived it in sharp

Edwardian and quasi-military executions, with high closings, lots of buttons and stovepipe or belled trousers. Then, in the mid-eighties, the power suit appeared with its big shoulders and blousy pants, and the double-breasted style reasserted itself again among moneyed Italianate dressers.

Single-breasted suits have also had their evolutionary ups and downs, with lapels going from superslim in the early sixties to superwide in the early seventies, with peaked lapels going almost extinct in favor of notched lapels, then staging a comeback in recent years. The jacket vent went extinct in the power-suit era, mimicking the perennially ventless Hollywood film silhouette. Vents don't film well. Then the British double vent returned to dominate.

Two or three buttons are always safe and reasonable. Four buttons or more tend to make one look like a sportscaster or a Vegas entertainer. But I have noticed that the higher-rolled three-button suits that were in fashion a decade ago, as opposed to three-rolled to two, are looking a little long in the tooth these days. Another jock-fashion pitfall. The three-button suit and the three-piece suit nearly disappeared between the seventies and eighties. But fashion won't let a good idea get away forever; it needs to change things up periodically and force some obsolescence on the male kit. Fashion is more motivated by economics than aesthetics.

Vests, called waistcoats in England, have been a part of a man's suit from the beginning. As a part of a suit, the vest was hard to find in the U.S. from the late sixties to the nineties, and I was delighted when they made a comeback. I think they were, for a time, a casualty of central heating, but then we discovered that actually they're very good for offices that can be overheated or overcooled, and today we need more pockets than ever, with the phone, the PDA, and iPod nano.

There are those who would have you believe that pleats are, once again, obsolete. I don't believe it. Big extreme triple pleats and reverse pleats are very nineties, but discreet pleats, especially on suit pants, are, to my mind, simply good engineering. They help you move and make it less likely you'll ever bust the ass of your pants. For trousers worn without a jacket, I did hop on the fashion bandwagon and wear flat fronts for their clean look, and I do have suits with flat fronts and they work fine. Maybe they look better when the jacket comes off, but pleats are a fact of life.

Cuffs—or turnups as the Brits call them—are strictly a matter of taste. Traditional guys usually go for them, but the old truism about plain bottoms making your legs look longer is probably true, and cuffs don't work on skinny trousers. Despite the trend for showing sock initiated by the visionary designer Thom Browne, I think a slight break at the shoe will remain proper until the end of the world. One of the biggest mistakes American men make is not wearing their trousers too short but having their overlong pants bunched up around their shoes. Jacket sleeves shouldn't be too long either. A half inch of shirt cuff should show with arms at rest.

One trick that off-the-peg customers can employ is to have a tailor open their jacket-sleeve buttonholes so that the buttons function. It costs about $10 per button, and it does give the impression of a bespoke garment. But nothing gives that impression like a good fit. Make sure you use that three-way mirror to check your fit. Perhaps the most crucial area of fit is in the back around the collar. The fabric should lay flat and not gather, and the jacket should fit snugly up against your shirt collar and not gap when you move. I always say you should be able to take a full golf swing or your jacket doesn't fit right. And don't just take the word of the fitter. Look at how he's dressed. Usually these guys are too long in the sleeve and trousers, just like most of their victims.

I was talking to Ralph Lauren about change in men's style not long ago and he took a really hard line that I agree with. He said, "If it doesn't look right now, it never looked right." Something to think about when you buy that suit. Shop for eternity.

ON SHIRTS

The shirt is the new suit. As we slouch casually toward apocalyptic informality this most elementary of garments has somehow inherited the mantle of propriety. "No shirt, no shoes, no service" is now the last frontier of civilization against urban nudity. It used to be that a man wore a suit. It was his uniform of status and civility. But now, leveled and humbled in the service of democratic regularity, we have devolved to a world of shirts and skins. If those are the choices, I know which team I prefer to play on.

"White collar" and "blue collar" don't mean much anymore. It used to be that a serious man wore the serious shirt, the white one. It marked him as management, an executive or professional, a man who worked with his head instead of his back. His shirt's whiteness and starched crispness proclaimed impeccability and authority. White gives the doctor or the scientist an aura of purity and gravity. It is the color of the most fearsome shark, bear, and tiger; the hue of the house-burying avalanche and the ship-crushing whale. It is the color of heat and the color of cold.

Take it away, Herman Melville:

"Is it that by its indefiniteness it shadows forth the heartless voids and immensities of the universe, and thus stabs us from behind with the thought of annihilation, when beholding the white depths of the Milky Way? Or is it, that as in essence whiteness is not so much a color as the visible absence of color, and at the same time the concrete of all colors; is it for these reasons that there is such a dumb blankness, full of meaning, in a wide landscape of snows—a colorless, all-color of atheism from which we shrink?"[1]

For the white man (or the white devil), this pristine shirt has served as the uniform of the ruling class. And although the small-jet executive has dandified himself in recent years, he still sports the white collar, even if the shirt's body is as blue as the stratosphere he inhabits. His collar is white in homage to his robber-baron predecessors in their detachable white boiled collars. The white collar also echoes the mystical investiture of prelates with powers beyond the mundane, and so the functionaries and minions of the corporate world still hold to the white shirt and tie as articles of faith in the elevation of the dutiful. The ambitious man still wears a white shirt.

On the lighter side, nothing looks sharper than the contrast of a white shirt with a dark suit when a man heads out for the evening. A man in a perfectly pressed white shirt looks, as Miles Davis would say, "cleaner than a broke-dick dog." White puts the form in formality, and if you're not dressed in a white shirt, you are not really wearing a tuxedo. White is right for night.

By day, we have options; more than ever, actually. The white shirt used to be a universal uniform for men—some stadiums cleared out the bleacher seats in center field because hitters couldn't pick up a ball coming out of all those shirts. But since today anything goes, a man chooses a dress shirt, a sport shirt, or a work shirt more on a whim than out of a sense of occasion. The sport shirt isn't really for sport, and the work shirt probably isn't for workers anymore; there's more likely a team jersey or a heavy metal T-shirt under the laborer's overalls. The denim work shirt is now the garb of the artisan—the vintner, the cheese maker, the high-end cabinetmaker—or the off-duty fatigues of the CEO, when he's off sweat-lodging with the board in his Panther Primitives tipi.

Dress shirts now come in many colors and patterns, and in the post-white-shirt era, businessmen's shirts are getting bolder in color and more daring in pattern. It's good to see men adopting audacious plumage. Why should humans be one of the few species where the female surpasses the male in hue and conspicuousness? In fact male drabness is cultural, not species related. American men may look boring, but in Italy and Britain the gents give the ladies a good run for their style money, and in some African tribes, like the Wodaabe, the men are spectacularly flamboyant, the real beauties. So, while I like white for night, I think a man needs to show his colors, and shirts can cover most of the wearable areas of the visible spectrum. The only chromatic caveats in shirt selection are related to skin tone. Colors that might sublimely suit my Hamite and Semite brothers do not always work with my pinkish Celt complexion.

Dress shirts come in many styles, usually determined by the style of the collar and cuffs. The most formal dress shirt has French cuffs that are folded double—giving the cuff more prominence—and closed by cuff links, the most appropriate form of gentleman's jewelry. Buttoned barrel cuffs are less formal, but they aren't incorrect except in formal situations. A tux needs links. Collars vary considerably in size and style. Some are dressy, some are casual, and there is a certain science to selecting a collar appropriate to the proportions of one's face, head, and neck.

A broad collar can balance a narrow face—think of John Kerry (why the long face, Senator?) or a lantern jaw—think Jay Leno. The obtusely angled spread collar is also a traditional Savile Row look, and it is the one collar that calls for a Windsor knot. Because of the way the collar falls when unbuttoned, the spread collar shirt doesn't work well without a tie. A spread collar shirt is a dress shirt or it's the wrong shirt.

The straight-point collar is acutely angled and it flatters a fuller or wider face. It was a good choice for Ted Kennedy or Tony Soprano. It works with a tie, or with the collar open, and it can also be fastened behind the tie with a pin or bar. Tab-collar shirts create a similar effect, pushing the tie up with a flourish. It never occurred to anyone that the tab collar could be worn without a tie until dandy Bob Dylan made tieless tabs all the rage in the sixties. It still looks positively Fourth Street.

The club collar, small and rounded, may be the hardest to pull off. With a face that's too big or too small, or tailoring that's not up to the task, it can look retro in a costumey way, making a man look like he should be wearing shirt garters and playing a banjo. But worn under a good face with natty haberdashery it can be a cool old-school look.

Nothing is preppier or more traditionally American than the button-down collar, which defines the Ivy League look. The style was intro-duced by Brooks Brothers in the "roaring nineties" (that's the 1890s); the buttons were originally intended to keep polo players' collars from flapping in the breeze. The button-down is not really a dress shirt, but most American men consider it such, and in the rube-trodden halls of Congress a white button-down and tassel loafers pass for dressed up. For years I believed that the button-down collar could not be worn with a double-breasted jacket until I saw Fred Astaire pull it off perfectly in *Yolanda and the Thief*. Of course Fred could pull off a necktie as a belt, but I tried the b.d. with d.b. myself and was surprised how fresh it looked.

Most American men wear big, baggy shirts that make them look even more schlumpy than their oversize suits do. I'm not sure if this is a side effect of the obesity epidemic or of the one-size-contains-all mentality of mass-market businesses. Also, American "trad" guys have long favored a loose, baggy aesthetic to differentiate themselves from their wasp-waisted continental counterparts. The Ivy League look was based on the natural sack suit, with no waist suppression, and the oxford-cloth shirts usually worn with this suit are sometimes described as "generous." Men of heft often think this stylistic generosity disguises corpulence, but in fact it accentu-ates it. A shirt should be trim and close to the body. The shirttail should-n't blouse out around the waistband of the trousers and the cuff shouldn't gape around the wrist, although it has been probably been cut that way to accommodate a wristwatch the size of a mini bagel.

Although European shirt makers generally cut slimmer, some of them alter their proportions for the American market. Charvet shirts sold in America are fuller than the Charvet shirts sold in Paris, although they are less full than the average American dress shirt. But things are changing, and even bastions of baggy like Brooks Brothers now offer slimmer alternatives.

My advice is don't rely on size numbers; try on the shirt. Yes, it's all pinned up and folded nicely, but don't be afraid to ask the salesperson to unwrap it for you. And if you love a shirt but it's too full in the body, a tailor can slim it for you, and sometimes the store will alter it for a few dollars more.

The worst male fashion trend of the present millennium so far may be the shirttail worn out. On purpose. I know that many consider it hip to go around with the shirt untucked, or even half tucked, like you slept in your clothes and haven't had coffee yet. I know this is intended to convey a youthful, casual je ne sais quoi, but more often than not it looks like he's too fat to tuck. Even worse than the shirttail out is when this is under a jacket. Of course some casual shirts are made to be worn out, and these have squared-off bottoms, but even these should not be worn under a jacket. A caftan would look better. Another egregious trend was unfastened French cuffs hanging loose through and far beyond the jacket sleeves, giving the wearer a waifish street urchin look. Accessorize this look with a tin cup.

Instead a man should pop those French cuffs displaying magnificent cuff links. At least a half inch of cuff should show beyond the jacket sleeve. If no shirt shows, it creates a sort of simian, knuckle-dragging George W. Bush-in-first-term effect. Better to err on the side of more cuff, like Sammy Davis Jr., and let it all hang out. Most men don't know what size they really are, which is why their shirts are too short in the sleeve and too tight in the collar. And many men, still growing when they should have stopped, try to hold on to their collar size like a treasured memory. Get a grip on yourself and get measured before your head explodes.

A man's shirt should always be fresh. Nothing else provides that finished look to your appearance. Send your shirts to the laundry. You may think you know how to iron, but that professional touch helps. Some men end the day looking fresh as morning; some, myself included, dishevel easily. If your shirt starts to rumple, change it and consider the benefits of light starching at the laundry.

Some men like to have their shirts monogrammed. This may be a deterrent to theft in a frat house, but I am content with the laundry mark inside the collar. I don't mind monograms when they are discreetly tucked away inside the jacket where they belong, but when I see initials on a French cuff across the poker table I tend to keep my derringer handy.

1   *Moby-Dick*, Chapter 42, "The Whiteness of the Whale."

ON TIES

I love the necktie because it is the only article of clothing in a man's wardrobe that has real enemies. Iranian revolutionaries, for instance, see the tie as an evil phallic symbol of Western decadence, emblematic of the Crusader's Cross of the Great Satan. The enemies of the cravat point to it as a symbol of conformity, even servitude. Some see covert obeisance to black magic encrypted in it, a fashion version of the "cable tow" of Masonic initiation rites.

The tie can actually kill the wearer, some tie critics point out—one reason it isn't worn on the factory floor. Others decry it as the only element in a man's wardrobe with no function—and so Silicon Valley tech companies tend to disdain it and some hard-line, form-follows-function devotees, like the management of IKEA, have banned it. But that's exactly what I love about the tie: its sheer, almost transcendental uselessness. The tie's only function is beauty, a quality of man that seems at low ebb in this benighted age. The functionless tie is to the wardrobe what the functionless soul is to the body. It is pure poetry. It is there for its own sake. It is an emblem of art and artifice. It is a flag without a country. And in the case of the long tie, it is an arrow, pointing to our manhood.

During my youth, neckties were required in many better restaurants, as were jackets. The "21" Club was a last holdout of this code, but in 2009 it too dropped the tie requirement for dinner (lunch had gone tie optional several years before). When I was a kid most restaurants had exquisitely horrible jackets and out-of-fashion token neckties available for boors who showed up lacking these requisite items, and it seemed as if these letter-of-the-law loaners were chosen for their blatant ugliness, to further punish the tieless for their temerity. But "21" had a beautiful plain navy necktie with a large "21" embroidered in red on it. I think these were discontinued because they were regularly pilfered. I wish I had stolen one myself.

Although many ties express membership or solidarity, like an old-school tie, a club tie, a regimental tie, or a silly tie emblazoned with donkeys or elephants, the tie can also express nonconformity. The hand-painted tie was in vogue in the mid-twentieth century. And we may see a group of men all alike in gray business suits and white shirts, but by their ties, if not their faces, we can tell them apart.

As the sublimely spurious-noble essayist Lord Whimsy wrote in *The Affected Provincial's Companion*, Volume One:

"One's tie, whether it is intended or not, proclaims one's personality (or lack thereof) in its color, pattern, material, and thickness; and yes, even one's choice of knot says much about what is afoot inside the bubbling noggin above."

The traditionalist declares his allegiance to all things Ivy with his rep stripes and arcane heraldica, meaningful colors and crests, usually pilfered from British schools, clubs, and regiments. The plutocrat favors large, glowing Italian ties of woven silk in bold geometric patterns (remember the power tie?) or repeating patterns of whimsical devices, from tennis rackets and golf clubs to Pierrots and death's heads. The bohemian tie is a tradition as old as the cravat itself. In the good old days ties were hand painted by the artists who wore them. There were Cubist ties, Vorticist ties, and Futurist ties. Avant-garde neckties were seen at Bloomsbury and the Cabaret Voltaire. The ties of the British artists sometimes resembled the camouflage of the Great War "dazzle ships," created by Vorticist Edward Wadsworth, while the Italian Futurist Giacomo Balla designed a necktie that was electrically lit. Photographs of Wyndham Lewis show him wearing scarves and neckties resembling the painterly abstractions of the Omega Workshops. Salvador Dalí not only designed ties for himself and for manufacture, but he also tended to wear more than one at a time.

It seemed that ties, in all their flamboyant uselessness, had the potential to serve as original works of art worn on the person. And so while the tie is often assumed by convention to express membership, allegiance, or solidarity; it is also capable of expressing absolute individuality and unrestrained eccentricity. Ironically the tie can simultaneously express both conformity and rebellion.

The fashion factor in ties has mainly to do with width. The rule of thumb is that a man's tie should be as wide as the lapels on his jacket. In the late fifties and early sixties, as modernism reached a sort of cultural zenith, men wore sleek suits with narrow lapels and narrow ties (the mode in fashion now). Then in the late sixties and early seventies ties began to grow wide again as a part of the Carnaby Street neo-Edwardian fop-a-delic aesthetic. Sergeant Pepper did not wear skinny ties. Excess was in the air and so were excessive vintage ties, which not only expressed the new camp sensibility but also happened to be very cheap. It is a general rule of fashion that things come back into fashion after they have hit the bottom of the vintage barrel and are adopted by poor but stylish youth, who are then noticed and imitated by fashion designers. One of the first promoters of the wide-tie redux was a young tie designer named Ralph Lauren. Then the tie didn't stop widening until it hit about five inches and the necktie pendulum turned again.

It's all about proportion. Slimmer suits need slimmer ties. The lobster-bib neckties from the eighties and nineties went with the NFL-shouldered power suits cavorting on Wall Street, glowering on NBA benches and dwarfing the talking heads in jock-pundit chairs. But the history of fashion is filled with regrets, and sometimes some of us can't go along with the pack. I firmly believe that there is a golden mean of neckties that will always be correct. Approximately three inches is the perfect tie and single-breasted-lapel width—permanently.

During the power-suit-power-tie aberration, I wore Hermès ties, because that luxury house didn't go wildly wide with the rest of the world but remained an island of moderation. I would also occasionally run into other well-proportioned ties at boutiques where a sense of modernism remained. Now that fashion has come back to its senses, I find many handsome, properly proportioned ties. A few years back, Brooks Brothers, in a rare moment of lucidity, introduced a three-inch tie under the University label. Then, in a moment of doubt, they discontinued them. But you can't fight public demand, and now that impeccable width is back at Brooks, a brand that once stood for the Platonic ideal.

For me, anything much slimmer than three inches is on the retro side, but narrow ties are now the fashion and that's OK. Men enamored of muscle cars and the Four Seasons (the group, not the restaurant) prefer skinny ties, and this is their prerogative if not birthright. It's good to defy the herd. A man should be prepared to hold out for life on matters of principle such as tie width.

But this is a moment, and who knows how long it will last, when fashion has dropped in for a visit with sanity. If it were up to me, ties would forever stay as they are this very moment, between two and a half and three inches wide. As for length, usually we are advised that the tie should reach the belt buckle or the waistband of the trousers. Vintage ties run short. This is because men's trousers rose higher on the body until the seventies, but also because men sometimes wore them short, almost like ascots. Today the Italians make really long ties. This is because they like to wear big fat knots, and that may involve a few extra loops around the knot. Too short is OK, too long is not. The last thing you want to do is get your tie stuck in your fly or pee on it.

In the matter of knots, there are many possibilities. In 1999 the Cambridge physicists Thomas Fink and Yong Mao published a book called *The 85 Ways to Tie a Tie*. The usual ways number about three: the four-in-hand, the Windsor, the half Windsor. I like the old four-in-hand because it's the easiest, as well as charmingly imperfect and asymmetrical.

On the subject of the Windsor knot, which may be the most popular knot in this age of OCD, I often quote Ian Fleming's *From Russia with Love* : "Bond mistrusted anyone who tied his tie with a Windsor knot. It showed too much vanity. It was often the mark of a cad." What I don't like, and what I think Messrs. Bond and Fleming didn't like, is the overly precise and symmetrical look of this knot and its overblown size. Aside from the cad, the Windsor is also the mark of the anal-retentive, the control freak, the nitpicker, the overfastidious, and the finicky. In the seventies huge polyester ties were often Windsor-knotted, and today we see the big knot flaunted by Italian dandies and other wearers of large, showy collars. I guess it's as close as moderns can get to a Shakespearean ruff. The Windsor is sometimes referred to as the "double military knot," and we've seen it on many drill sergeants and state troopers, not to mention General Patton and Adolf Hitler. The Windsor knot has its place, and that's with a spread collar, but it's not the all-purpose knot. The four-in-hand, however, is what one would call devil-may-care, creating the welcome impression that you got dressed without looking in the mirror. Casual asymmetry is the charm of the four-in-hand. It goes with the flow and no two are alike.

In my capacity as wardrobe adviser to the nation, I have received far too many queries on the tie dimple. Men seem to obsess over it. I just put on a fairly thick silk tie from Timothy Everest and tied it up with my usual four-in-hand and it came out with a double dimple, and I thought it looked good. But it just turned out that way. I like that kind of natural process. Creativity often owes a lot to accident. When it comes to your tie, just tie it.

The Bow Tie

The bow tie, except as the pasta known as farfalle, declined in popularity steadily over the second half of the twentieth century, and in this century it has become almost controversial. Writing in *Slate*, one Rob Walker called the bow tie a "stunt accessory" and "the nose ring of the conservative." Considering the gift-wrapped look of rightist pundit Tucker Carlson, I could almost agree, but that would assume the bow must always be neat and prissy. It can also be tousled and askew, a protest against the rising tide of conformity, and I have to stick up for it. I am a bow-tie wearer, maybe only once or twice a month, not counting black-tie season when it is de rigueur, but there's nothing sissy about it. If it comes to a brawl you're safer in a bow than a long tie.

Some men seem actually afraid of bow ties. *Dress for Success* author John T. Molloy is bow-tie horrified. He wrote, "If you wear a bow tie, you will never be taken seriously, and no one will trust you with important business." So much for Winston Churchill! I suppose some sub-urbane Americans do think, He wears a bow tie; maybe he's a Communist. Well, Karl Marx did wear one, but it's really about suspicion of those who choose to be different. Bow-phobia became so extreme in recent years that the traditional black bow tie with a tux was frequently eschewed at the Oscars in favor of a black four-in-hand—perhaps the worst trend in men's evening wear since the tux with a turtleneck of the sixties.

Maybe the decline of this noble form of neckwear started with ex-haberdasher President Harry Truman, a bow-tie wearer who dropped atomic bombs on two largish cities. Or maybe bow-phobia stemmed from a subconscious fear of natty, neat, and determined Black Muslims, as personified by Malcolm X. Or maybe it was fear of Pee-wee.

Once the mark of the urbane, devil-may-care personality and worn by such heroes as Bogart and Sinatra, the bow tie began to connote the opposite type. By the seventies, it was seen as the mark of a nerd or geek. Think of Jerry Lewis in nutty character or Mayberry's spooked deputy sheriff, Barney Fife, or Pee-wee Herman and presidential candidate Paul Simon—nerds, albeit men of courage under their less-than-formidable exteriors. But the bow is coming back. They don't like it? Good! If you have swagger, a bow tie can be a badge of courage.

There are also many practical advantages to the bow tie. It won't droop into your soup or get caught up in the cogs of machinery, so it's a good choice for men of action. It must not be too large—the mark of a clown—and it must be hand-tied carelessly. The anal-retentive clip-on look is the sign of a compulsive hand washer or a potential Unabomber. It looks like it might squirt water or suddenly go for a spin. But a beautifully asymmetrical, slightly tousled bow is a perfect look for a nonconformist man of style. It's best as an alternative, not a uniform, but it has a legitimate place in our repertoire.

The Ascot

In automobile advertisements, we often see subtitles that say PROFESSIONAL DRIVER. DO NOT ATTEMPT THESE MANEUVERS. Perhaps pictures of men in ascots should carry a similar warning. The ascot is tricky. Some men wear it effortlessly, while others will look pretentious no matter how they wear one.

The true ascot is a double-knotted tie worn with a pin as part of formal daywear. It is named for Ascot Heath, in England, a famed horse-racing track where the Royal Ascot race has been a showcase for fashion plates since 1711. What Americans commonly refer to as an ascot is a foulard, a sort of neckerchief usually worn around the neck inside one's open shirt collar to dress up a casual look. Once a chic accessory for informal occasions, this ascot is now a rare sight. When one is sighted, it is often considered a mark of affectation, ostentation, or foppishness. Once sported regularly by stylish men such as Fred Astaire and Cary Grant, the informal ascot somehow came to be associated with annoying people—harmlessly pretentious men like Thurston Howell III of *Gilligan's Island* and Dr. Smith of *Lost in Space*. Or harmfully pretentious men like Mobutu Sese Seko. But worn by a relaxed man with nothing to prove, the ascot, or neckerchief, still works its charm. It adds a more civilized touch to an open shirt collar than does a T-shirt or a thatch of chest hair. I like to wear one when I'm entertaining at home. Somehow wearing a tie at home seems odd, but a scarf or a foulard ascot knotted simply around the neck, worn low so it peeks from under the collar, adds a nice touch of color or pattern to a simple outfit. It shows more care and respect than an open collar, and it also shows a certain bravery—I dare to care.

The Scarf

It'll do the tie job when you don't feel like wearing a tie. Like *mes amis Parisiennes*, I dig scarves even when it's not cold, like in May or June when there's a cool evening breeze. It gives you that je-ne-sais-quoi feeling, *non?* Especially a colorful piece of cotton voile or batiste or a silk foulard as a finishing touch. I used to wear a kaffiyeh occasionally until an old lady slugged me in a café. I guess she thought I was Hamas—now I just wear my colorful Omani kaffiyeh, which nobody thinks is political.

A scarf subs for a tie in casual situations. It's good for impromptu stick-ups or dust storms, worn like a bandanna. Arterial bleeding? You've got a tourniquet. Bad-hair day? Wrap your head like Little Steven. Or tie it loosely and wear it under an open collar so we don't have to look at your pec fur. Blind date? You've got a blindfold. And a scarf under the shirt collar always provides that urbane élan, bohemian verve, or sporty pizzazz that helps get you through the doldrums of the day.

ON SHOES

If the shoe fits, they say, wear it. If the shoe fits, I say, try the other one on.

Asymmetry is fundamental. Most of us have one foot bigger than the other, and this alone can be a good reason to have shoes made to order. Nothing a man wears is more important than his shoes. They are his primary vehicle—his platform, his conveyance, his limo, his racer, his getaway car for the feet. More than any other item in the wardrobe, shoes are tools, functioning as a necessary extension of the body. They are also clues to the mystery of life.

The thirteenth Duke of Bedford, who wrote a swell twentieth-century update of Thackeray's *Book of Snobs*, noted the significance of the shoe thus:

"A head waiter once told me: 'I can always tell people by their shoes. People who are only trying to show off and impress you wear fabulous clothes but are not prepared to spend a lot on their shoes.'"

My advice is to spend freely on your shoes. You have only one set of feet and expensive shoes will last almost as long as you do, provided you get them serviced, as you would your other vehicles. Excellent shoes won't go out of style, unless you have shopped while not in your right mind. Expensive shoes will also help you last longer—at least your feet, legs, and spine. And being comfortable in your shoes should make you happier and more cheerful and thus more magnetic and sexy.

Like that head waiter the duke spoke of, most people who appreciate the finer things will notice your fine shoes, even if you are wearing 501 jeans and a Hanes white T-shirt. And they will think, Here is a man with his priorities straight.

Of course, if you do embark on the bespoke shoes course and have lasts made of your feet (after which the price per pair goes down), you will have shoes in the image and likeness of your feet. Making your feet, in a way, godlike. So make sure that these shoes, which cost as much as a serviceable second car, are always well taken care of. If you buy your shoes readymade, as most non-billionaires do, it's prudent to do some research in order to discover what foot "fit model" your feet most closely resemble. Every shoe is made for someone, and if you can find a maker whose ideal foot resembles yours you will be comfortably shod.

The great dandy Beau Brummell polished his shoes with champagne—that is, he had his man polish them with champagne—but I don't imagine the valet popping corks in the morning. No doubt the task was performed with the dregs of the night before. If you find yourself with some leftover bubbly, why not try a Brummell shine yourself? It's probably nothing special, but it will give you something to talk about. Many men like to shine their own shoes. Veterans seem to have a thing about it. I refuse to shine my own except in case of emergency, since the bootblack is one of our endangered professions, like stonemason, Morse code keyman, or hot typesetter. Yes, farriers still do well taking care of horse's shoes, but how easy is it to find a good shine for one's oxfords today? This is unfortunate because the professional shine is generally far superior to what the do-it-yourselfer can accomplish with his liquid shoe polish. Pro shines can still be found in many train stations, airports, and shoe repair shops, and they are probably the least expensive luxury.

Today many young men have problems dealing with shoes because before hitting the job market, they never really wore them. They lived in sneakers since toddlerhood. Which is, I suspect, one reason that the fashion-forward periodically tell us that it's OK to wear sneakers with a suit. Maybe if you've been embezzling and the auditors are in the office, sneakers will give you an edge if you make a run for it, but basically sneakers with a suit is a fundamental error, no matter how much the sneakers cost or who designed them. Would you wear wingtip brogues with a Knicks uniform?

Sandals are heavenly. My kid calls them Jesus shoes. I wear them around the house in the country. Usually I wear them with socks to save people the trouble of looking at my feet, which have had it a lot rougher than the rest of me. There is a school of thought that it's really square to wear socks with sandals, especially, for some reason, Birkenstocks, a practice that apparently suggests you are a Communist college professor, but in casual situations, why not? Sandals with socks can even be worn with a suit, especially if you are a Communist college professor.

Flip-flops, however, are never to be worn with suits; in fact they are not to be worn outside the home, unless you have a swimming pool. They look sloppy and in some situations creepy. If you wear them on the street and there's any justice, you'll step on a pop-top and blow out that flip-flop.

Flips-flops are actually designed to prevent you from catching athlete's foot in the locker room, not for strolling the boulevards or climbing mountains. Recently I was descending a stone staircase approximately a thousand meters to a favorite seaside restaurant in Capri when a man blew out his flip-flop—not on a pop-top but on a sharp rock—and nearly tumbled to his death. When I warned him of the dangers of flip-flops he just shrugged. Flip-flops are fool shoes.

My grandmother was an archconservative when it came to men's clothes. Among her decrees was that in the evening only white shirts and black shoes are proper. Once she caught me heading out on a date in a pink oxford button-down; she said that if I showed up to pick up her daughter looking like that she wouldn't let her go out with me. That was OK because her daughter was my mother, who is totally not my type, but she did have a point. Evening should be dressier than daytime.

Of course going home to change for dinner is a bit of a luxury these days, and in an age when good restaurants are filled with men in Air Jordans, we can hardly complain about a fellow in a pair of brown calf brogues, can we? Still, raising the bar is a tough job that somebody's got to do.

There are also those traditional sticklers who state unequivocally that brown shoes are not to be worn with a blue suit. This is one of those old rules that no one can remember the reason for. If the shoes are dark brown, why not? Brown shoes have been worn with navy blue by U.S. Navy aviators since 1913. There are also those who state that wearing brown shoes with a black suit is improper, and I have to agree, although why you would be wearing a black suit in the first place is another question.

White shoes, or partially white shoes like spectators or saddle shoes, are a traditional part of a gentleman's warm-weather wardrobe and society has long observed rules for their seasonal wear, particularly in the American South where you may be ostracized as a vulgarian for breaking seasonal taboos. (Picture little old ladies aghast at Tom Wolfe.) The usual dictum is that white shoes—and white trousers and suits—are to be worn only between Memorial Day and Labor Day.

These are two relatively recent holidays in the scheme of things (adopted in 1866 and 1882, respectively). Alternatively Easter has been cited as the appropriate beginning of white-shoe season instead of Memorial Day, and as Easter is a movable feast celebrated on the first Sunday after the first full moon following the vernal equinox, theoretically the white-shoe season could begin as early as March 22. Memorial Day is the last Monday of May and Labor Day is the first Monday in September, meaning that a strict white-shoe season could last as few as sixty-three days or as many as 138.

This rule seems kind of silly in the twenty-first century, given the overwhelming evidence for global warming and the fact that Jerry Seinfeld wears white sneakers all year long. I think if we're going to have a rule about it, it should be that white shoes are to be worn only in baseball season, meaning from early April until the beginning of October. (If your team makes the play-offs or the World Series, of course, you will be granted a white-shoe extension.) Or if you don't follow baseball, you may wear white from All Fools' Day (April 1st) until Columbus Day.

Men wearing shoes of unusual hue are sometimes assumed to be entertainers or pimps. But to give evolution some leeway, I suggest that it's time to let men explore nearly the full spectrum of footwear. Colored shoes are a much easier way to express one's anima than wearing a skirt. I myself have two pairs of blue shoes, one pair of green, and two pairs of plaid shoes. I see no reason why the male of our species should be less colorful and splendid than the female, although hue and tone should be managed with regard to occasion. Never wear blue shoes when asking a man for his daughter's hand in marriage or red shoes when applying for a loan.

Loafers are for loafing. Somehow, during the barbarian revolution of the last half century, loafers have asserted themselves as quasi-dress shoes. The typical congressman probably considers penny loafers or tassel loafers and a white button-down shirt to be a dressy look. This might be OK for a prepster to wear to chapel, but many men desperately hold on to boyhood for life. There is a widespread belief that tasseled loafers are dressy shoes, no doubt because of their Eastern college heritage. They are for class-conscious loafing.

The Japanese have also had a hand (a foot, really) in the rise of loafers as companions to the business suit, since they are always taking off their shoes. But the Italians have also perpetrated some particularly ugly low-vamp loafers that show far much too much sock and are favored by wiseguys. Loafers are not dress shoes. They should be worn with a suit only when one is off duty and peacocking it. For formal business, like weddings, funerals, depositions, and trials—such as O. J. Simpson's, during which bloody Bruno Magli loafer-prints were entered into evidence—loafers should be avoided like contempt of court.

By the way, I am totally in support of the Asian custom of removing one's shoes indoors, particularly in the home, as it helps keep out microparticles of dog shit and its resident organisms, tar and motor oil, mud, sand and gravel, among other undesirable substances. Should you choose to adopt this mode of living, which I believe will one day be universal among the civilized, it's best to have some slippers available for guests, some of whom will have holes in their socks.

In Western regions of the United States one often sees cowboy boots worn with a business suit or other types of clothes not usually associated with ropin' and wranglin'. I am often asked if it's OK to wear cowboy boots with a suit. If you asked me "Is it acceptable to wear a turban with a business suit?" I would answer "Yes—if you are a Sikh." So if you are a Texan or a cowboy or you play one on TV, you can wear boots with a suit.

Lately we see lots of guys in driving shoes—you know the moccasins like Tod's, with little rubber nubs on the soles and moving up the back of the heel—walking here and there, nowhere near their Lamborghinis. These shoes say, "I'm rich and I'm not walking very far." They work for some people, and they do come in a nice spectrum of colors. But as a purist, I really think you should own a sports car to wear them, or at least be driving a stick, and they should never be worn in the backseat.

ON SOCKS

"Both of your socks should always be the same color. Or they should at least both be fairly dark."

—Dave Barry

Some men call it hose, but we might call them "hosers." A real man wears socks. And he wears good socks. Skimping on socks is a sure sign of a cheapskate. Socks should be luxurious and in good repair. Actually socks are one of the cheapest items to which the idea of luxury can be attached. A fifty-dollar pair of socks can make you feel like a million bucks.

For some reason, though, socks often confuse men. The question I have been asked most in my capacity as an alleged expert on such things is, "Should my socks match my shoes or my trousers?" The answer is neither. But if we had to choose one it would be the trousers, because some contrast between shoes and socks avoids the appearance of wearing booties. But there is no reason to match socks to trousers except, perhaps, on the most formal or serious occasions when we are seeking a little formality or even severity.

I always advise that socks should freelance, perhaps picking up a color cue from another item in one's apparel, such as the tie or shirt. Matching the shirt was a favorite Fred Astaire tactic, but socks can also match your sweater or your eyes or your 1969 911 Targa. It's not necessary that they actually match anything. It's fine for socks to go their own way. You can feature independent socks, like argyles, as long as they're in the same spectrum as the rest of your gear. If you're wearing a suit, the socks can echo the color of your tie or pocket square. Or they can be another color altogether, as long as it matches the rest of your look in tonality and subtlety. There's no reason at all for socks to be a solid block of color. I wear navy socks with small white polka dots, brown herringbone socks, wildly striped socks, and black socks with small red devil heads on them. They add a little spark on those rare occasions where I'm wearing a black suit. At least I won't be mistaken for a priest.

I have been taken to task on this subject—one reader suggested that I go to Bergdorf's and speak to a fashion consultant about color matching. This fellow was sure I had broken a rule. Clothing does not have rules the way golf has rules. It has principles based on aesthetics. I will grant you that if you are giving the State of the Union address and you are wearing a navy suit, a white shirt, and a red tie, as most good commanders in chief do on such occasions, you probably will want to wear navy socks, not red ones. If you wear red socks while giving the State of the Union address, some will peg you for a Communist and insist that the vice president take over immediately, citing the "unable to perform" clause.

The point is, we have to use our good judgment. If I'm going to the loan department at the bank, sure, I'll likely wear gray socks with my gray suit, but if I'm going to the racetrack I might try to match my socks with the green in my tie. Right now I am wearing an orange shirt, khaki pants, and argyle socks with gray, brown, and tan in them. I am so happy with this combination, my ankles might explode. And I certainly will explode before I consult a consultant. This isn't science; it's art.

I have also been criticized on occasion by women who feel that men should never, ever wear white socks. This is an overreaction to the Fonzie-esque greaser look of the fifties, where white socks often intervened between pointy black shoes and blue jeans. But today if a man is wearing white shoes or white trousers, white is a fine choice. And this is where hose comes in, meaning thin, fine-quality socks. White athletic socks should only be worn with actual athletic shoes during athletics or work boots while doing physical labor, and tube socks should only be worn when masturbating in someone else's bed, or better yet, never.

Cotton socks don't have to be thick. I have some beautiful fine-gauge cotton hose from Charvet in Paris and I recommend this style highly because it doesn't shrink like wool, and if your housekeeper is anything like mine, you have wool socks that you have passed on to the wife and/or children. Incidentally, I don't believe that one size fits all. Even in condoms. One-size socks cause holes, or cause you to find your sock heel on the sole of your foot around the talus bone.

The feet have their own commandos, and we notice that sockless-ness has seasonally reached epidemic proportions. More and more men are wearing socks less and less, on more formal occasions and deeper into the fall.

I have friends who rarely wear socks with their shoes, ever. I remember the photographer Peter Beard going sockless under his Weejuns in the depths of winter, but I always thought this had less to do with style and more to do with manhood rituals such as picking up a hot frying pan bare-handed. Photographer Wayne Maser rarely lets socks come between his beautiful bespoke suits and his beautiful bespoke shoes (which are, in an almost brutal gesture of je ne sais quoi, unlaced). My superbly turned-out amigo Hooman Majd usually goes sockless through the summer and perhaps past the autumnal equinox.

I have noticed that for a few summers now the always daring *GQ* editors have been wearing shorty socks (aka footies or loafer socks) with their summer suits. In recent years I've loosened up on the subject of these almost-invisible socks, which my mom wore and called "peds." I first saw them on men on the golf course (somewhat surprised they passed club muster), and after several seasons of ped persistence I've stopped suggesting to guys in my foursome that they wear the ones with the pom-poms at the heels. Now I notice that these sockettes are big with the sneakers crowd. I should probably confess that even I have been entertaining breaking down and getting some peds in the interest of avoiding a mid-calf tan line. I mean, as Miles Davis said to Roland Kirk, "We all got to change." And shorts are legal on the course now at Winged Foot. Maybe next year.

I am a sock person. You'll usually find me wearing them when my brethren are going sockless. This is partially a matter of personal style, but I am convinced that wearing socks is healthier for my bog-trotting Celtic feet. I also think going sockless works better in the country than in the city. It is not a good business look unless one is in the creative or lifeguarding sector. The city is a gritty place and socks are protection against the dog-trodden, rat-shat, sooty streets. Then again, I'm out there on the sidewalks craning my head at girls in strappy sandals. (Sorry, darling!) Maybe I'm a hypocrite. Or maybe it's just my dank Irish feet.

Foot notes

1   Good socks should be washed inside out. Trust me.

2   Foot odor can be caused by socks that are not absorbent, so all synthetic socks should be avoided. That said:

3   Purity is a virtue in many things, but wool socks are not one of them. Often, a small amount of Lycra or other material is added to the blend for elasticity and to help the socks retain their size and shape through laundering. I would not consider pure wool socks unless I had a laundry staff.

ON HATS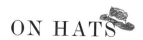

If you are a boy, you must wear a cap. If you are a man, you must wear a hat. Your hat is your crown. Without it you are a humbler, commoner sort. Without it you lack a fine tool of chivalry. John Barrymore said the only reason he wore a hat was so he could take it off in front of ladies. Doffing it also salutes a flag or conveys respect. Donning it keeps your head warm. It makes you taller. It centers your aura. It cushions your brain. It gives you something to talk through or throw into the ring. The hat is such a personal friend; we wonder how it ever managed to disappear from the gentleman's quotidian kit.

The last forty or fifty bareheaded years are a historical aberration. Hats were always assumed to be an indispensable part of a gentleman's wardrobe, at least until the sixties. The myth is that John F. Kennedy killed off the hat by attending his inauguration bareheaded. In fact, he wore a topper to the swearing-in and it was sitting on a chair when he gave the speech that kicked off the New Frontier. It is true that Kennedy was not a hat fan and that he went bareheaded much of the time. Too bad, a good stiff bowler might have deflected that fatal shot or at least hindered the aim of the gunmen.

Another theory on the hat's hiatus has it that, after years of wartime military service, men became sick of wearing hats, but men have been serving in the military forever. I suspect that the hat's disappearance was actually a by-product of the dawning of the Age of Aquarius, and the consequent down-to-there hair, shoulder length or longer. The Beatles and The Stones did wear the occasional chapeau, but basically the freak flag flew free in the breeze during that decade of stylistic revolution. Proud manes refused to be contained. The hat was, finally, old hat.

But hair has ebbed again, and now it seems once more that a man needs a hat to be fully dressed. It's not only a way to top off a look with truly personal style, it also helps protect against ultraviolet radiation and falling objects and it can be used as a screen or disguise when anonymity is desired. Fezzes and turbans can be dramatic, but a brimmed hat is eloquent and its adjustments can express or even conjure a mood.

Brim snapped down in front shows that the hat is in a serious, hard-boiled film-noir mood, à la Sam Spade or *The Thin Man*. Brim up signifies a light, screwball-comedic, Joel McCrea/Fred MacMurray/Gene Kelly kind of attitude. Brim way up in front and way down in back signals a spunky outlook like that of Mugsy of the Dead End Kids. Brim swept to one side, a look Johnny Depp seems to like, means you're eccentric, idiosyncratic, and bohemian. Tipped back on the head à la Belmondo, the hat signals self-confident ease. When I'm feeling artistic or rebellious I might wear the brim down all the way around like the British painter Wyndham Lewis, or wear the brim all the way up like the German artist Joseph Beuys, who wore a fedora indoors and out. Brims are made to be adjusted. Consistency is the hobgoblin of the hatless.

Stick your ticket stubs or a press card in the band for extra edge. Wear straw in summer, felt in other seasons. Black looks charmingly dangerous; gray is elegant and goes with anything; navy is deep and dressy; brown is rich and uncommon. Other colors are true rarities that set you even further apart from the anonymous crowd. I have a few hats, like the pea-green

Worth and Worth fedora and the violet Borsalino with brown grosgrain brim trim, that are real works of art. And if you're really impressed by them you can say, "My hat's off to you!"

Happily we've noticed that the hat has definitely revived in recent years, at least among artists, rakes, swells, dandies, and other sartorially adventurous men. After years of disuse by hatless hordes, the fedora is, at this point, as attention-getting as a tattoo and it comes right off with no residue. Maybe Don Draper, the sex-symbol hero of television's retro-fest *Mad Men*, is keeping something under his fedora. A secret, perhaps, that he doesn't even know himself. Hats have magic. It's how we top it all off.

There was a brief vogue for the fedora during a cinema-generated nostalgia wave in the eighties when men took to wearing what they unfortunately called "Indiana Jones hats." Harrison Ford did look fine in a hat, but his imitators were less impressive and the marketplace was flooded with subpar felt. But the fine hat was never entirely extinct—there was a hat-wearing underground throughout the uncovered years. I know, having been part of it since the seventies, and I've had plenty of fedora-wearing friends, from musicians like August Darnell to directors like Charlie Ahearn to artists like Joseph Kosuth. But I never minded being the only hatted man in the crowd. The way I wear my hat? Oh, no, they can't take that away from me.

I wear many hats. I like that they symbolize how many different jobs I do. Most of them are fedoras—the most classic and modernist of men's hats—but I suppose the star hat of this present fashion moment is a variant on the fedora called the porkpie. The porkpie hat is the mark of the determined hipster, the kind of cat you might see hanging around a jazz club or a pool hall, maybe wearing a button-front leather jacket and pointy shoes. It's a Tom Waits, Johnny Thunders kind of hat. It has a narrower brim than a fedora and a flat top with a circular indent. Usually the brim is worn up. It is often worn with a goatee, soul patch, and/or toothpick. The porkpie is associated with the great saxophonist Lester Young (for whom Charles Mingus wrote "Goodbye Pork Pie Hat"), as well as Thelonious Monk and Dexter Gordon. Now the short-brimmed porkpie is raging again, thanks to Pete Doherty, the singer-songwriter of the British bands The Libertines and Babyshambles and noted both for his liaison with Kate Moss and his misadventures with controlled substances.

I'm seeing more hats than ever on the streets: fedoras, porkpies, Tyroleans (the tweed short-brims), Irish walking hats (also tweed), "newsboy" or "golf" or "Ivy League" caps—both Irish style and Sicilian style—and rainproof oilskin bucket hats. I have hope that the hat and the proper cap will kill off the plague of the baseball cap as casual sportswear. Turtle of HBO's *Entourage* can continue to wear his baseball cap backward or sideways or inside out, but more and more men are replacing that clichéd cap with something that isn't logoed or licensed or redolent of the silent style-free majority.

And with the hat revival just beginning, there's plenty of unexplored territory at the top. As a huge generation now enters its distinguished-years phase, the venerable homburg beckons. My grandfather always wore a gray homburg. It is a crisp felt hat with a hard brim turned up all around and edged in grosgrain ribbon that matches the hatband. My grandfather always drove a Cadillac because its ceiling was high enough to drive while wearing a homburg. Traditionally homburgs were worn by mature men and were often favored by diplomats, bankers, serious capitalists, and other distinguished types. It was popularized at the turn of the twentieth century by King Edward VII of England, a portly gentleman who was nevertheless a great trendsetter. (He also popularized the dinner jacket, the trouser turnup, and leaving the bottom vest button undone.)

There's the derby or bowler, once the uniform hat of the British middle class, which is often associated with such diverse characters as John Steed of *The Avengers*, Laurel and Hardy, Alex, the thug of Kubrick's *A Clockwork Orange*, and Oddjob, the Bond villain whose bowler was a lethal weapon. This once very popular hat had virtually disappeared, but it has been sighted lately on such diverse men of style as Jack White of The

White Stripes, Jakob Dylan of The Wallflowers, and rapper Nate Dogg. Being very crisp and sturdy, its use could catch on for its value as a crash helmet or protection against nightsticks—which is why it was once a favorite of toughs such as the notorious Plug Uglies of nineteenth-century Baltimore.

Lately I've seen hats showing up in all the trendy boutiques. Someday the men who buy these may discover serious hats. The majority of my felt fedoras come from the estimable Worth and Worth, an institution that has been a New York tradition for seventy years. A few years back, when hats seemed to be going the way of the passenger pigeon, Worth and Worth moved out of their prime location on Madison Avenue and moved into a space on the third floor of an apartment building on East 55th Street. I thought that soon I might have to fly to London to get my hats blocked, but now that hats are back, Worth and Worth is moving to 57th Street, on the second floor, and is hopefully soon headed for street level. When I do go to London I always stop in at Bates of Jermyn Street, an ancient hole-in-the-wall chock-full of magnificent lids. Fine hats are also made by Borsalino of Alessandria, Italy (established in 1857), and Christys' of London (established in 1773).

Many men's hats have a feather stuck in the band. It is my experience that usually the feather would have been better left on the bird. Another interesting detail of the hatter's art is the elastic band and grosgrain-covered button found on some better hats. This is a wonderful old feature. On windy days you can put the button inside the buttonhole on the lapel of your suit or overcoat, and if your hat is caught by the wind the elastic band will catch it before it can be run over by a taxi or you are run over chasing it.

Here are a few important pointers about hats: When they get messed up, take them in to get blocked. Take your hat off when you are indoors, unless it is an indoor area equivalent to outdoors, such as the subway or an airport. If you don't, according to my grandmother, you will go bald. Always tip your hat when meeting a lady, when passing a church or when a funeral procession passes. Always remove your hat during the playing of a national anthem, even if you do not support the regime. And never put your hat on a bed. It's bad luck. Don't ask why. When you have nothing to do you can put your hat on the floor and toss a deck of cards into it, one at a time. There is no good reason to do this, but it will teach you a thing or two about life and how the cards fall as they may.

HOW TO HAVE A STYLE

"Style, neurologically speaking, is the deepest part of one's being, and may be preserved, almost to the last, in a dementia."

—Oliver Sacks

Style is what you can't forget.

That's why they could prop up Willem de Kooning in front of a canvas when he couldn't feed or wipe himself, and he could still turn out de Koonings, whether or not he knew they were de Koonings or who de Kooning was. Style runs deep. It is in our very DNA, like a fingerprint but much more entertaining.

What is style?

It so distinctive yet it's hard to pin it down. Some say, "If you have to ask, you'll never know." Others say, "I know it when I see it." Talking about God, whom Picasso probably considered a peer, the randy Cubist said, "God is really only another artist. He invented the giraffe, the elephant, and the cat. He has no real style. He just goes on trying things."

Style isn't about trying things. It's semi-effortless. George Clinton of Funkadelic said: "If you've got funk you've got style." Perhaps George Gershwin expressed it best in Zen-like lyrical form: "The way you wear your hat / The way you sip your tea / The memory of all that / Oh no, you can't take that away from me."

Style is something so deep in our manner that we may not notice it in ourselves. It's deeper than our memory. It cuts to the bone but it floats near the ceiling. It's metaphysical. But everyone who knows you remembers it. It's our visual and behavioral signature.

Style is the way Clark Kent took off his glasses. The way Jean Cocteau rolled up the sleeves of his suit jacket when he read *Le Monde*. The way Bill Evans slumped over the piano so his neck was parallel to the keyboard. The way Louis Armstrong played the cornet with a handkerchief draped over it—perhaps like Buddy Bolden did, so nobody could cop his fingering. The way Muhammad Ali shuffled. The way Michael Jordan wore his shorts. The way Cary Grant rolled his eyes. The way Sinatra held a cigarette. The way Patrick Ewing wore a T-shirt under his jersey. The way Jackie Gleason said, "And a-way we go!" Style is something that can't be taught. It's something that can't be lifted or copped. It's something essential.

The bad news for many is that they have no style to live on beyond them. If you are a type, you lack style. Style is unique and ephemeral, and to have a noticeable style, in art, speech, dress, sport, or physical carriage, your manner has to be unique, or at least a rare thing. In my childhood, people complained that it was an age of conformity, but now we have entered the age of the clone. Why imitate if you can duplicate? Now even nonconformity has become clichéd, with rebels rolling out of the alternative assembly line, decked in designer rebel uniforms, with tattoos selected from a brochure and piercings in the usual shocking spots.

Great stylists might be imitated, but they can't be co-opted because their combination is locked in. And if their followers and enthusiasts put some real work into it, they can transcend imitation of their idols and come up with a riff or stroke of their very own. Some of the most stylish people I have known have been called phonies, and maybe they started out that way, but by the time they got up a head of steam they were *real* phonies, that is originals; the training wheels of imitation had fallen off and they were freewheeling. Affectation can take root. It can sprout wings, if it's taken to heart. We don't start out as Oscar Wildes or Oscar Madisons overnight.

Style is in the details, in the nuance. It's not a fashion statement. At best it's not even a statement; it's a phenomenon. It's a practice, a study, a form of research. How can I wear this shirt the way it's never been worn before? It can seem arch, if not well done, but it's a creative process. Some art stinks.

Style is partly innate, but it is also cultivated. Style comes from a combination of personality, study, and work. You're born with some style tendencies, the way a young baby has personality right out of nowhere, but then you have to develop it; you have to practice it and refine it to have a style worth calling a style. And if you don't use your gifts, that style will evaporate and you won't have a style anymore, just a bunch of mashed potatoes.

You cultivate a style through work, even if it sometimes looks like play. You practice the things that you have to do in life until you are contributing something to the way they get done. Your style might even begin as an error that suddenly looks good or sounds good and you know you're on to something. If you have style, the way you speak contributes to language—it makes the ineffable effable. If you have style, the way you dress contributes to the landscape of civilization, and the way you bob and weave or shake and bake contributes to the game, taking it to the next level. Sometimes cultivation takes, sometimes it doesn't. But once style takes hold it becomes part of our being and it grows like a beard.

Style is the opposite of fashion. The *Oxford English Dictionary* defines fashion as "conventional usage in dress, mode of life, etc., especially as observed in the upper circles of society; conformity to this." Fashion is imitative. It's about belonging, being in with the in crowd. Style is what sets a man apart from the crowd or attracts a crowd. Real style comes from within; it's the visible component of your character and personality that you place in the world outside you.

Style is about setting yourself apart, being unique and authentic, being what the stylish Sam the Sham called "in with the out crowd." That professional paragon of style Noël Coward said, "I have never felt the necessity of being with it. I'm all for staying in my place." Your place is your own being. Baseball hitters talk about "staying within themselves." Having style is staying within yourself. It's about the way you work. To riff on the hitter's metaphor, it's about "working the count," how you deal with what's thrown at you.

Style is different. If we hear something from a sax or see something made by a pencil and recognize it as new, that's style. Wyndham Lewis said, "The best artist is an imperfect artist." The perfect artist is finished. He's done. He has found it; he's not looking for it. The genuine stylist is too caught up in developing and applying his modus operandi to the job to rest.

Style can be how you draw, how you play the cello, how you write, or how you dance, but it can also be how you speak and how you tie your tie. Style isn't taste. As Lewis said, "Taste is dead emotion, or mentally treated and preserved emotion." Style is spontaneous emotion; you feel your way through the world. You dig for it, you find it, and you put it out in the world.

I guess it's what Smokey Robinson called "the way you do the things you do."

"How do you do?"

"Splendidly. How do you do?"

HOW TO BE FORMAL

As the world has become smaller and more homogenized, as tribes trade their beads for cK T-shirts and folk costumes are abandoned for thirdhand GAP and the jungle drums are stilled by Lady Gaga, we seem to be making a last-ditch, desperate show of individuality. We collect tattoos like prison lifers, we grow sadhu beards, pierce our ears like the Tlingit and our noses like Berbers, and scarify ourselves like the Yoruba, while dressing in distressed costumes influenced by outlaw motorcycle gangs, lumberjacks, mountain men, Ostrogoth armies, and Druid conjurers, and somehow we don't even know why. Suddenly, in a new millennium, we are prefab rebels without probable cause. Never have the normal looked so weird.

Men say they don't like suits and ties because they want to be comfortable and they want to be themselves. They say that suits are for the regimented, so they'll wear a mass-manufactured exact copy of a coal miner's jacket from the nineteenth century in the hope of feeling different, authentic even. But as Anne Hollander points out in *Sex and Suits*: "when all men wear a white tie and a black tailcoat in the evening, the individual character of each man is made more important, not less."

This is the true nature of formality. Dressing in the same mode for an occasion does symbolize cultural allegiance, but at the same time it accentuates our own unique characteristics. Today, formality, that secular sacredness of yesterday's society, is nearly extinct. When you go to what was once a formal black-tie affair, you may still see a good number of men in tuxes and others mimicking a tux in a black suit and white shirt, but the mob will be a motley of whatever. There are suits, sport coats, Ramones T-shirts, NFL jerseys, blue jeans, and tracksuits. There simply are no dress codes anymore.

Anything goes. There is something truly decadent in this lack of social solidarity. The idea of occasion has vanished. Looking at the gorgeous harmony
of a chic nightspot in a Fred Astaire movie, I feel like the Romans must have
felt with barbarians running through the gates. Surely this is the nadir. What
can surpass this in disorder?

Now if the code had broken down in a real quest for individual freedom, I'd be OK with it. But in fact it has broken down out of craven fear.
As Hollander declares: "Dressing up is more risky than dressing down, too
much respect for the occasion is considered worse than too little."

I believe fervently that we have to get back to the dress code and that
bygone sense of ritual and occasion. It is political, in a subliminal but very
real sense. We must dare to overdress. We must turn away the shoddy at
the door. We must have the courage to look as uniform as a symphony
orchestra, in order to give back to individuality its context. And so it is my
sworn duty to always dress like I have somewhere better to go later.

First rule: black tie means you have to wear a tie. And it should be
black. Duh. And make that a bowtie, please! An occasion that calls for dinner clothes is not the time for creativity. This is as close as a civilian gets
to the uniform of a hero. Wear it proudly. It is the uniform of a gentleman.
The tuxedo, properly worn, leaves plenty of room for brilliance, wit, and
improvisation in the details and within "the rules of the game."

In the early-to-mid-twentieth century, "formal" meant white tie, full
dress, tails. But there are very few occasions that still call for this standard
of formality. Even President Obama, who has a natural sense of formality,
didn't have the heart to go for white tie at his own inaugural ball, attempting instead a compromise with a tuxedo and a white tie. So we might as
well admit that it's all over. I'm probably not going to need a tails suit again
unless there's a revolution. (Or I win the Nobel Prize.) But it does seem that
there is a distinct revival of black tie afoot. Maybe it will help pull us back
from the brink of anarchy and barbarism. If it doesn't, at least we'll go down
the tubes looking sharp.

In recent years we have seen a lot of goofy improvisation at black-tie events. Some guys think it's cool to show up in a tux jacket and jeans and maybe cowboy boots. On Oscar night we see all sorts of "creative black tie" —black shirts, long ties, no ties, open collars. We are seeing attempted tuxedo mutation, with notch-lapel black suits trying to pass themselves off as tuxedos with satin or grosgrain lapel facing. A real tux has peaked lapels or a shawl collar and its pockets are double besom without flaps. A real tux has striped trousers. (White-tie trousers have two stripes.) Tux trou do not have cuffs.

Some events call for "black tie optional." This simply means that the people throwing the bash would prefer that you wore a tux, but they don't want to dissuade guys who don't have one or are afraid of wearing one from buying a ticket. If it's optional, exercise the option: wear a tux and look better than the rest.

A single-breasted tux or dinner jacket requires a vest or cummerbund. Some of my hep, young colleagues believe the cummerbund is obsolete, but it's not. It's actually more important than ever because we live in an age of low-rise pants, and we don't want white shirt showing through under our jacket button. Although both options are correct, many men prefer wearing a vest with a single-breasted dinner jacket because its angularity matches a peaked lapel and because a vest helps keep your linen under control. A cummerbund seems appropriate with the curved lines and the more at-ease silhouette of a shawl-lapel jacket. If you wear a double-breasted jacket, you don't need a vest or cummerbund.

Vests raise other issues, however, so they should be chosen with care. A black or white vest, perhaps with some texture, can add verve and individuality to a tuxedo, but unfortunately the majority of evening vests I encounter seem inspired by riverboat-gambling fashion. I'd rather look like a waiter than Doc Holliday. Vests shouldn't resemble upholstery. They should be seen and not heard. The same goes for cummerbunds. Adults should resist the temptation to relive their proms in matching-pattern bowties and cummerbunds. There are well-dressed men who wear colored vests, and when the color is a quiet one, it's hard to argue against it. Still, call me a fogy, but I think color takes away from the conceptual elegance and restraint of black and white.

Again, the only really proper black tie is a black bowtie. It may be straight edged or a butterfly; it may be skinny or fat. Personally I like a big fat bowtie like the Duke of Windsor's or a skinny one like the kind Hugh Hefner wore on *Playboy's Penthouse*. The tie should be of the same material as the facing on your lapel. A bowtie should not be tied too perfectly and symmetrically or it looks uptight. This is why clip-ons should be avoided, although pre-tied ties can be OK. Charvet makes beautiful pre-tied bows that strap on. The only acceptable clip-on is the one that twirls or squirts water.

Tuxedos are black, but sometimes the best black is really blue: midnight blue. When Edison's light bulb replaced the candle, the black tuxedo suddenly appeared a bit greenish. Apparently this discovery was made by the Duke of Windsor: a very dark blue looks blacker than black in artificial light. Lighting might have improved since then, but midnight blue is still an excellent choice.

In the winter a proper black overcoat should be worn over a tux. A Chesterfield with its velvet collar is an appropriate choice. A tan raincoat is not. A polo coat makes you look like a delinquent frat boy. A man should have a proper black overcoat for tuxes and cold-weather interments.

Dinner jackets can also be white for wear in the summer or in the tropics. Usually they are worn with the same black trousers that go with a black jacket. And usually cummerbunds are preferred with white jackets because they're cooler than vests. Some men like to wear a white mess jacket instead of a white dinner jacket. A mess jacket is a short, waist-length jacket inspired by military formalwear. Although it is double-breasted, it is not meant to be fastened. It looks like a tails jacket without the tail. Mess jackets are still worn on full-dress occasions by the military. White mess jackets were a really popular look for civilians once upon a time, and they still look great on someone lean and fit.

There are two main styles of tuxedo shirts, the turndown collar and the wing collar. The turndown collar was almost universal until the nineties, when there was a big return to the retro wing of the old Gay Nineties. The wing collar, a stand-up collar with little triangular wings, is standard equipment with white tie and an option for black tie. The wing collar does not look good on a man with a fat face or a short neck. I think it is actually hard to pull off a wing collar with a tux today. Most wing wearers look like poseur tux renters. But if you dare, take care that the wings do not cover the bowtie. Incidentally the idea of wearing a long tie with a tuxedo is one of the worst sartorial trends of the modern age. It's the mark of a coward. A tux calls for a bowtie.

Tuxedo shirts may be pleated (the test of a good laundry) or have a piqué front. Ruffles, along with pink, gold, or lime green tux shirts, are best confined to the Las Vegas stage. We certainly wouldn't tell Tom Jones not to wear a ruffled shirt. It frames his chest hair so nicely. But there's an exception to every rule, pussycat.

Tux shirts invariably have French cuffs and usually they are closed in front with three studs, one area where a man can show off. Studs are the bling of the discreet. I also like a placket-front shirt that hides the buttons, presenting a totally closure-less front. There is a school of thought that a man should not wear a watch with a tux. I can appreciate that. Who cares what time it is at a ball? (Except Cinderella.) But a dressy, thin watch is forgivable. Unlike a diver's watch, which should get you tossed overboard.

Shoes usually mark the difference between a tux renter and a tux owner. A renter often wears his black business shoes. If he's a poor dope, these may even be black wingtip brogues. Clunky shoes are no good. Black calf plain-toe lace-ups are acceptable. Oxfords in patent leather are welcome. Sometimes these can be rented too, but sometimes rented patent leather shoes look like they've been bowled in. Black calf opera pumps—with or without a bow—are appropriate. Belgian shoes, a light, slipper-like shoe with a little bow on the vamp, were my default black-tie shoes for years. But whatever shoes you choose, they should be sleek and light, the better to trip the light fantastic in.

Then there is the smoking jacket. The French call a tux "Le Smoking," even if you can't smoke in it in France anymore. The smoking jacket, like the tux, was originally intended for dinners at home, but it has taken to the streets. Often these are made of velvet and come in rich colors. In the sixties there was a color explosion in dinner jackets too. When I was a stand-up comic I favored a bright green or a silver sharkskin dinner jacket. I think these helped me get laughs. I drew the line, however, at ruffled shirts. Pleats are for dandies; ruffles are for Tom Jones, pirates, or potato chips.

Nothing finishes a tux like a fresh carnation. But please eschew the salad greens and the bud vase. A proper tux has a thread behind the buttonhole for the express purpose of keeping the boutonniere in place. Incidentally, there is a tuxedo maker called After Six, and that is because tuxedos are meant to be worn after six. Wear it before six and you may be mistaken for a maître d' on his way to work.

Someone once asked me if tuxedos were out of style. He said a woman had told him that men now wore black suits instead. I said, "Tuxes aren't out of style; they *are* style." When I see a man in a black suit at a black-tie affair, I always feel a little sorry for him. Every man should have a tuxedo. It is the sartorial expression of elegance, even hope. I have two tuxes because I'm always hoping something comes up two nights in a row. And maybe someday we will all dress for dinner again.

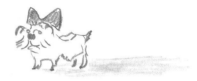

JEWELS AND THE MAN

I have never felt the urge to wear earrings except on Halloween or at one of those specialized theme parties where the ladies wear the pants and the fellows, um, stuff their shirts. I suppose there can be a piratical rakishness to a certain type of fellow with a ring in his ear and a gleam in his eye, but mostly earrings seem like a big mistake.

The only thing tackier than a signing-bonus diamond stud on a dude is two of them. I understand that some guys feel the need to gild, gaud, and bejewel themselves, but that's what watches, cufflinks, studs, and tie bars are for.

I guess some men have ancient instincts and haunting déjà vu to deal with. Maybe they were kings, chieftains or witch doctors in former lives. Maybe they lived in a nomadic pre-banking, pre-interior-decorating society in which one tended to wear all his wealth on his person in case a hasty change of scenery was required. And I suppose that an argument can be made today for upholding a tradition of street aesthetics. Pimps have flaunted bijoux for generations (Do pimps come in generations?), perhaps because ladies often have eyes for precious stones.

And magic may have something to do with it. I don't really want to delve into the metaphysical properties of minerals in this chapter, but we do know that idols once capable of eliciting hallucinations of deities (according to Julian Jayne's *The Origin of Consciousness in the Breakdown of the Bicameral Mind*) were often studded with jewels, particularly in the eyeball area, and sometimes in the mouth. I recall that Mick Jagger once had a large emerald set into his smile; this stone allegedly emits a powerful healing ray, yet its mystical power did not preclude the gem from being repeatedly mistaken for spinach.

Restraint is a gentlemanly virtue. We all have a yen to show off once in a while, but are not yens sometimes there to be resisted? In fact, being subtle and restrained is simply a higher form of showing off. Jewels are for the class that says "classy" a lot. They're street status, but they won't get you into the country club. As a Thorstein Veblen–quoting theorist of the leisure class, I like my jewels inside the watch movement. It's about inconspicuous consumption. In an age of obscene business practices, the point is less about the demonstration of your disposable wealth than the demonstration that you are not a criminal or a vulgarian.

Cufflinks are enough for me, but maybe that's because I'm wearing a shirt. I suppose if I went around bare-chested like 50 Cent or in a T-shirt-based costume or a pornographer's plunging neckline, I might dig necklaces. There certainly is some appeal to the atavistic Barbary Coast dandy aesthetic of Keith Richards or the late Brian Jones or the fictional Jack Sparrow. I can see the charm in a string of shark teeth or doubloons. Sometimes a guy needs a shot of mystique.

Even I have been known to wear a chain with a medal on it. I like St. Christopher, especially since the Vatican pulled his license, and I actually have a little thing for the Miraculous Medal, not so much out of devotion to the B.V.M. but just because I like the idea of a miraculous medal. It's a reminder that you can do just about anything if you try hard enough and get a few breaks. And I like goddesses in general—from Athena and Hera and Artemis to Santa Magdalena. But I wouldn't leave my shirt open to have the ladies ogled by the public. If I wear a medal it's for my inspiration only. Medals, crosses, scapulars, stars of David, and the red strings of kabbalah or Tibetan Buddhism are all best worn secretly under our profane threads.

Let us create a value system of inconspicuous consumption, based not on scarce and precious commodities but on wit, fetish, and imagination. Instead of bling, let's flaunt cheap things, like beaded surfer bracelets that cost a dollar. I don't like those silicone bracelets—they just remind me that athletes use performance-enhancing drugs—although I'm OK with Stephen Colbert's red "Wriststrong" or the black "Livewrong" bands.

A gentleman's jewelry is his cufflinks and his watch. Cufflinks are usually thought of as dressy, but there's no reason that you have to be wearing a suit and tie to wear them. Sometimes we need a little punctuation to our look, and cufflinks do that job. Cufflinks have more to say than buttons. They are the periods and commas, exclamation points and question marks of our wardrobes.

Silk knots worn on French cuffs give you a chic spot of color. But cufflinks can also convey symbolism. I've got ancient Greek gold coins with satyrs on them—the mark of the satirist. I've got a hand-painted set depicting gambling, booze, and women. I've got sterling golf balls, Deco enamels, recycled manual-typewriter keys. I even have a modernist pair designed by Prince Sigvard of Sweden that I consider art. Why waste a chance to say something?

The watch is jewelry with an excuse. We do need to know the time, and the wristwatch is a more elegant timepiece than a BlackBerry or an iPhone. Today's watches are interesting for their indulgence in complex obsolete technology. A watch that costs as much as a luxury automobile doesn't tell time any better than a $20 Casio digital watch. In fact, the prohibitively expensive watch probably doesn't have a calendar, stopwatch, or alarm that plays *Für Elise*. The luxury watch must be wound, unless it winds itself. But that's the point. A man can buy a box that will keep all of his self-winding watches wound, just in case he doesn't have a yacht that rocks. But the watch reverses the usual paradigm of value—the more work it is to use, the more effort that goes into achieving the result, the more valuable it is. It's almost about reverse efficiency.

As with other luxury items of conspicuous consumption, the watch is often about the brand and the rarity of the model. But the market has become so complicated that many of today's watches are strange hybrids, like a watch that owes its basic design to sports performance, specifically skin diving, mutated by encrusting it in diamonds. The pseudo–sports watch has become the dominant genre of male bling because of its hockey-puck-like size. Watches get bigger and bigger, approaching the parody proportions of Flavor Flav's alarm clock. What's more pretentious than a guy in a sharp suit, crisp linen and a three-figure tie in a giant watch that lights up and is guaranteed to a depth of 660 feet? Down there on the ocean's floor it might still be ticking, but the wearer won't be. That's an icon of surplus utility, like a 200-miles-per-hour speedometer, the sure sign of a man with too much cash. Less is more, now more than ever. I always thought it was cool that my friend Gene Pressman wore the ladies' version of the Rolex Oyster because he thought it more discreet.

Sports watches should be worn for sports, or at least when you're wearing sports clothes. And isn't there something slightly creepy about watches that give you too much information? Do you need to know the phase of the moon? That's useful for lunatics perhaps. The month? If you can't remember that, a watch won't help you much. The time in Chicago? I'll bet it's usually Miller Time. The truth is that your phone or a $50 watch can do everything a $50,000 watch can, except show everyone you're a big shot. I want a watch with no features.

A better way is to very quietly and reluctantly admit that you are a big shot, though it means very little to you and is even a bit embarrassing. That's why a proper luxury watch is slim and discreet, poking out occasionally from a crisp cuff and giving people a peek when you reach across the table or check the hour.

Generally jewels are better off in the hands of the ladies. The dames wear vanity better than we do, having had centuries extra of practice, and maybe they are better equipped to handle the mystical aspects that surround the extraordinary value and aesthetic appeal of jewels. A late woman friend of mine, a jeweler who was very much into crystals and the inherent properties of stones both semiprecious and precious, once made me a golf charm for my key ring, which she claimed would improve my game. It was made of gold wire and a big, round, green stone. The first time I carried it in my pocket, I had the highest score for eighteen holes that I could remember. I wondered if the thing was cursed, but then it occurred to me that she was probably didn't know that the point of golf was to score fewer points. I put it in the drawer where it sits today. Maybe I should try it for bowling.

Jewels require discretion, which is why I'm wearing seventeen jewels right now, all hidden inside my watch.

ON BELTS

"He couldn't see a belt without hitting below it."
—Margot Asquith on Lloyd George

Ah, the belt, man's first garment. Invented, perhaps, by Adam himself. Inspired by a snake. Man wore the belt long before he wore the pants, long before the toga or tunic. The belt held up the fig leaf or the codpiece. Man stuck his knife under it, or a bone. And as form follows function, millennia of multiple garments followed the good old cinch, the anchor of the wardrobe.

The belt retains its ceremonial primacy, at least in the warrior class. Wrestlers and boxers don't win crowns; they win belts, big gilded, emblazoned bands of glory. And in the East, one reckons a warrior's degree of deadliness by the hue of his sash. If you could wear only one thing, a black belt would be a good choice.

I think the very first joke I was ever heard was this, told by my grandfather: "Why does a fireman wear red suspenders?"

After I thought about it for a while he delivered the punchline: "To hold his pants up!"

That's how we learn about life. From somebody trying to confuse us. But I also realized there was a certain underlying truth. The fireman indeed wears red suspenders to hold his pants up. And in New York, I believe New York's Bravest wear black suspenders to hold up their big, heavy, waterproof, flame-resistant pants.

For most of my life I have worn a belt to hold my pants up. Sometimes it was a skinny "continental" belt a half inch wide with two buckles. Sometimes it was a thin black belt with metal studs on it manufactured by an off-duty Hell's Angel. Sometimes it was a one-and-three-eighths-inch-wide cowboy belt with a big buckle made of hand-tooled leather or woven horsehair. But most of the time it was a seven-eighths-inch-wide black or brown calf belt with a nondescript silver-, gold-, or brass-toned buckle. Why? Because sometimes one doesn't want to make a big display of holding one's pants up.

Suspenders, once universal menswear, are today almost an endangered species, but one does still see them on natty, sartorially confident men. Oscar Wilde decreed that trousers should hang from the shoulders, and the literate tailor Alan Flusser agrees that suspenders provide the very best trouser fit. In fact the wise Mr. Flusser decreed, "There is simply no place for belts in the realm of tailored clothing." He points out that they disrupt the integrity of the suit and "they are particularly disruptive when one is wearing a vested suit."

So what happened to suspenders? They went out in the two belt booms following the world wars. It is theorized, reasonably, that men got used to wearing belts while in uniform and didn't want to go back to hanging pants when they put their civvies back on. But there's also the matter of trouser length. In the old days the pants met the suspenders halfway, around the navel. Today's low-rise trousers, instigators of plumber's butt, don't work well with suspenders because basically the hips have to hold them up anyway.

I have given up on both belts and suspenders by having my suit trousers made with side tabs for adjustment. I don't mind suspenders, although I do tend to associate them with Wall Street wankers who wear comedy suspenders—somehow these fellows reek of desperation. An even sadder look is wearing suspenders with trousers that have belt loops. Those empty loops look so lonely and useless. And the worst offense is wearing suspenders and a belt simultaneously. That's what you call profound pessimism.

If you want to wear what Americans call suspenders and what the Brits and those who admire them call braces, and experience the true difference between trousers and pants, have the loops omitted from your trousers and have them made with a proper rise, where the waist is considerably higher than the au courant at-the-hip stance, and with an English or fish-tail back, where the braces buttons are elevated above your seat. The result may look odd at first, but under a jacket it will be sublime. Properly tailored trousers that hang from the shoulders create an effect entirely different from trousers hung from the hips. They are draped elegantly and move with fluidity. Tango, anyone?

Americans love cowboy gear, and the cowboy belt is one of the classic accessories, a favorite of brush-clearing hicks and brush-clearing hick presidents. The cowboy belt is often hand-tooled with friezes of Western lore, accompanied by big and showy buckles handcrafted of silver or bronze and studded with turquoise and other semiprecious stones. In some arid and lonely regions of America, this is the epitome of the visual arts. Sometimes the belt is further festooned with double silver loops known as keepers and a silver tip. This show of pelvic flamboyance is undoubtedly intended to draw attention to a bulge in the pants of the sort that led Mae West to remark, "Is that a pistol in your pocket, or are you just glad to see me?"

For some wranglers, a big silver buckle and silver tip protector are not enough and so shiny silver "conchas" are applied to the belt. Conchas are usually roundish silver ornaments of American Indian heritage, riveted to the leather. They may be stars, skulls, iron crosses, spades, hearts, clubs, diamonds, or silver dollars. Conchas have no function other than decoration, providing traditional bling and an aura of roguish danger. Think Jim Morrison or the increased chances of getting hit by lightning.

The Easterner's version of the flashy belt is the plaque belt buckle, a plain silver rectangle suitable for engraving. The buckle can be monogrammed, and that detail made the belt popular in the early twentieth century. My friend Andy Spade wears a plain calf belt with just such a classic, unassuming silver buckle; his is quietly engraved "LOSER." So much more amusing than those street-vendor jobs, like the curious "Boy Toy" belt Madonna sported in early middle age.

The Western belt was made extra wide to hold up America's blue jeans under challenging conditions such as bronc busting, bull riding, tie-down roping, and tarring and feathering. But for many Americans, especially the hip-hopping denizens of the inner cities and their worldwide imitators, the belt has been dispensed with and pants are held up as if by magic or willpower. Jeans seem to levitate with no visible means of support. I see youths walking the streets of New York with their pants covering perhaps half their underwear, held in place as if by surface tension.

This "pants on the ground" look has been around for a decade or so now. It seems to be a rebellious fashion, intended to alienate a certain segment of the population through the defiant display of undergarments while mystifying others through the sheer defiance of gravity. I see young men walking down Broadway literally holding up their pants by hand. I believe this fashion has its origin in the jailhouse, where belts are traditionally taken away from inmates to prevent them from hanging themselves (and presumably others). I assume suspenders and garters would be similarly impounded, should a white-collar criminal have the temerity to report to the hoosegow so attired.

I have seen pants perched so precariously on the hips that I suspected Velcro was involved in their levitation. Perhaps the real meaning of the flaunted-underwear phenomenon isn't about the jailhouse but is related to Chinese foot binding, high heels, and hobble skirts. Just as long fingernails proclaim a woman doesn't work with her hands, and certain fashions exist as proof that labor is physically impossible when so dressed, so flaunted underwear demonstrates that the wearer doesn't need to move quickly. I wonder how many young men have been apprehended by belted gendarmes because of their unsecured britches—giving literal meaning to "fashion victim."

Fortunately this fashion seems to be on the wane, and we needn't fear for the belt's future. Besides keeping pants up, belts can add flair to a casual look. The silk-ribbon belt was popularized by British dandies who wore the colors of their regiment or club, and it has been a preppy favorite for decades. Fred Astaire took this look and ran with it, using his colorful old neckties as belts. I also like the classic braided belt, which is made of thin, braided strips of leather or horsehide, in a weave similar to that of huarache sandals. This belt is infinitely adjustable, not stopped every inch as a conventional belt is; the prong of the buckle can slip into the weave at any point. The most useful belt I own is reversible calfskin, black on one side, dark brown on the other; the silver buckle swivels, making it the perfect accessory for the traveling man.

The logomania that has gripped fashion for several decades has resulted in a variety of branded buckles. I wouldn't wear the classic Hermés "H" buckle myself, but it's fine on my friend Hooman, or for that matter on any Harry, Henry, Hank, Horace, Hector, Hassan, or what have Hugh. The same goes for Gucci's "GG" belt, which really works best for men like Gilbert Gottfried, Glenn Gould, George Gershwin, or Graham Greene.

The web belt started as military gear and crossed over to civilian popularity: tough, woven cotton with a brass or chrome buckle and tip. It's another analog belt that's infinitely adjustable. Then there's the venerable leather military belt with a strap that reaches up over one shoulder, known as a Sam Browne. The belt's namesake was a British officer who commanded a regiment of Punjab cavalry in Lahore, in what was then India in the First War of Independence. Captain Browne lost his left arm in action, and this made it difficult for him to draw his sword; the addition of a shoulder strap to the traditional garrison belt relieved that problem. The design caught on, particularly because it could accommodate more weaponry. It's still popular with state police and police states, as it provides support for pistols, ammo, mace, pepper spray, nightsticks, and walkie-talkies.

In his spring 2008 collection, John Galliano went military-belt crazy, showing all kinds of web belts, from basic Sam Brownes to a full-on George W. Bush–on-the-flight-deck, crotch-framing harness. If Galliano is to be believed, men of the future will add belts with abandon, strapping on all sorts of electronic devices, carrying cases, canteens, and manteens, just because they look tough. Maybe it's a visionary fashion move. I hate the look of cell phones, beepers, and other devices hanging from a dress belt. If you must hang gear from your belt, then wear a belt designed for the purpose. Batman and Robin never wore their Brooks Brothers belts on the job; they wore the Batman utility belt, which accommodated a radio, a camera, a flamethrower, night-vision goggles, acetylene torch, stun grenades, burglar tools, tranquilizer darts, first-aid kit, bat-light, batarangs, bat-cuffs, bat-lasso, bat-taser, bat-heater, bat-saw, cash, and presumably a black American Express card. The bat-belt was also very impressive looking.

Extravagant belts were prominent elements of many ancient wardrobes; they kept blousy clothes close at the waist, where a man of action hinges. Whether sash or cincture, the belt drew the eye toward a zone both erogenous and divine. Today the cummerbund, descendant of a waist sash adopted by British colonial officers in India, survives as a relic of the ancient flash of the sashed when worn by traditionalists with black tie. The word comes from the Farsi *kamarband* meaning "waist closure." Although it's often omitted from the tux ensemble today, when worn properly it can serve as a visual slimming device, making the legs look long and lithe.

The sartorially savvy blogger Mordechai Rubinstein is a belt aficionado, seeing its division of the body in two as a heightening effect, making both short and tall men appear taller. He also finds a Talmudic significance in its bifurcation of the body, "to ensure that 'one's heart does not see one's nakedness.' While our fashion has changed radically," he continues, "many communities have retained this custom. That's because it's considered a sign of respect and eagerness to 'gird our loins' with a special belt before we stand in front of G-d." The philosopher is also practical; he finds the belt a necessity in this day of digital burdens and tight pants.

ON UNDERWEAR

Underwear should remain under the pants until it's time for it to come off. This is why it's called underwear. The flaunted underwear look that seems to have migrated from the cell block to advertising agency creative departments is not a fashion for gentlemen. If I can see your underwear you *will* be arrested some day, if I have any say. That means back to jail, where this look started and belongs. (For more on this subject, see the previous chapter, "On Belts.")

Another outré sub-trouser strategy is called going commando. This means eschewing undergarments altogether. Apparently this usage derives from the Scottish phrase "going regimental," which means following tradition by wearing nothing under one's kilt. Other theories suggest that soldiers have often dispensed with underwear to relieve themselves more easily on the field of battle and to avoid "crotch rot" in damp, tropical theaters of war.

Most offices do not offer comparable conditions, so men who go commando in the urban environment are engaging in covert nudism out of some obscure macho impulse that they themselves might not even understand. It's not worth it, boys. Underwear makes sense for many reasons. It reduces abrasion on the intimate and private parts that might come from zippers, heavy woolens, or rough seams. It protects the organs of propagation. It prevents skid marks on the Super 120s. It is, in short, emblematic of civilization.

Many of my correspondents remark that they went commando to "feel free" and comfortable. These freedom-loving commandos should recall the words sung by Kris Kristofferson and remember that "freedom is another word for nothing left to lose," and usually the contents of our shorts are among the things we do have left to lose and would definitely rather not. I cannot imagine how going without underwear could be more comfortable, unless one also dispensed with trousers. Think of the scratchy wool, the cold, cruel zipper, the blue jeans's seam.

Freedom is one thing, but flopping around is another. And I remember thanking my underwear in high school on occasions of spontaneous wood. Underwear helps a man control involuntary spontaneity as well as what side he dresses on. Jeans and other snug pants leave no doubt as to the gender or mood of the wearer. And is not package display the very point of skinny jeans? This is expected. We are roosters, not capons.

Observe the breeches worn between the Restoration and the Regency era. We know precisely how Napoleon was hung and on which side Brummell dressed, and there's no shame in that. It is said, if you've got it, flaunt it—and for those with it, flaunting can be done with some discretion. And for those not with it, there's always the Spinal Tap zucchini prosthesis.

Tight pants, including jeans, require briefs not boxer shorts. Boxer shorts, which cover but don't cling, are for wear under trousers. And yet boxers, big boxers the size of NBA shorts, are often chosen by those who like to display underwear in public. Go figure.

Some women indicate a preference for boxers on their men, but they aren't the ones wearing the pants. In recent years we have seen the increased availability of trim-cut boxers that won't bunch up under modern man's tight pants, a good compromise.

As a guy that men complain to about such things, I have heard rumbles about irritation caused by elastic waistbands. Brooks Brothers still makes very old-school "French back" and "tie back" boxers in white and oxford blue. They have three buttons in the front and employ buttons or a drawstring in the back to fine-tune the size. These shorts are handsome and rather figure flattering and entirely elastic free. I'm not big on "lingerie" for men, but if I remember correctly, I once had this ancient style ripped from my body. She must have been a fervent traditionalist.

Men who are cheap often skimp on their underwear because it won't be seen, except perhaps by significant other(s). This is foolhardy, because as women know, when one is in the barely dressed mode it's best to look especially good. A man who wears cheap or worn underwear under an expensive suit is not to be trusted. He has a bad attitude toward himself, defining himself by how others see him and not how he sees himself. Wear the silk shorts of a king, the Egyptian cotton of a pharaoh.

ON PHYSIQUE

America is a nation of fatsos and anorexics. Or manorexics. We lead the world in obesity, actually doubling the global average. The rate of obesity in America is ten times that of Japan, the land of sumo. What's it all about? Do we think we can push the world around with all that heft?

It used to be that everybody was pretty lean. If you look at old movies, especially documentaries that show real people and not actors, fat people were quite rare. Today two out of three adults in the United States are overweight. The situation is similar in Britain, the world's leading consumer of fast food. Why the change? Is it the proliferation of hamburgers, fried foods, and all-you-can-eat pasta? Is it the drive-in world that has reduced the need to walk? Or is this gratuitous growth a symptom of some deeper metaphysical hunger eating at people, making them eat?

Are the new fatty fundamentalists storing up calories for the "end times"? Are they readying for the Rapture in case lunch won't be served? Whatever it is, the ballooning of humanity is a riddle bacon-wrapped in a glazed mystery inside an enigma with a side of fries and a large, corn-sweetened cola.

The Department of Defense has called obesity a national security issue, as apparently twenty-five percent of military-age young people are too fat to serve (that's nine million of them). It makes me feel for the peace-freak kids of my generation who defected to Canada to avoid serving in Vietnam. They could have just defected to Dunkin' Donuts.

Decades ago, in any crowd there'd be one fat kid called Tubby and one skinny kid called Skinny. Or maybe the fat guy would be called Skinny and the skinny guy Tubby. Now, of course, such nicknames might even be illegal. We aren't supposed to notice, even when we're squeezed into a corner by a pack of grazing behemoths.

That's partly because of fat liberation. Such groups as the National Association to Advance Fat Acceptance and the International Size Acceptance Association tell us that fat is fine; it's normal. Hey, it's beautiful in its own way. They say that discrimination against fat people is a form of "lookism," in which people are judged by their attractiveness according to preconceived notions of beauty. One of the most activist groups that I have encountered in New York City is a cabal of morbidly obese people who agitate for wheelchair ramps and accessibility in restrooms, not because they've been wounded in wars or crippled by infectious disease but because their eating habits have put them on wheels. They roll into mayoral campaign events and wheel around the sidewalks toting signs, lobbying for wheelchair accessibility everywhere. If the obesity lobby continues to be successful, we can envision the sidewalks of New York being replaced by conveyor belts.

Of course, the obesity boom is not all about gluttony. It is also about poverty-related malnutrition. Once upon a time, poor people were skinny. Today, the obese are generally from the lower end of the economic scale. Many overweight people have been denied the opportunity to eat properly. Poor neighborhoods lack good grocery stores and restaurants. Fruits and vegetables can be difficult to find. And the poor suffer from widespread "food insecurity," meaning that they often don't know where or when their next meal is coming from.

A hundred years ago, being fat was a sign of wealth and status. Today, it's the just opposite. "You can't be too rich or too thin" has been attributed to Wallis Simpson, the Duchess of Windsor. Now, of course, we know that you can be way too rich and way too thin, sometimes even at the same time—what used to be called "the ladies who lunch" became the "social X-rays." But a duchess couldn't make that statement today without being charged with promoting eating disorders. That's because anorexics and bulimics are literally fashion victims. Many of them fall into these delusional diseases because fat is despised by those who would be chic.

In the old days a guy would go to a fashion show, meet a model, and want to buy her a drink. Today he wants to buy her a club sandwich, milk shake, and fries. Many of the fashionable starve themselves, some fight food cravings with drugs or cigarettes, and some have their stomach stapled, all to appear sleek and svelte. In the beginning it was mostly women who were given to soul-searing battles with weight, but now men too have embraced the cult of skinny with a vengeance. It wasn't long ago that muscles were required. Models sported big pecs and guns, massive lats and boulders, and the *Men's Health* "six-pack" was essential. But in recent years, that look became as de trop as Fabio. The men's runways have been dominated by the least dominant males: skeletal wimps, scrawny nerds, gaunt dweebs, and wasted weenies. They're here, they're mere, and they're in fashion. Fortunately, a healthier role model seems to be returning, thanks to the recent outdoorsman fashion and the accompanying beards that require a more manly physique to pull off. And manly physiques, in their own arena, seem to get manlier and manlier.

We've been through the lean years, and the cut look of the juiced body-builder is as old hat as Arnold Schwarzenegger. Who knows what the future will bring? In the NFL, four hundred pounds is the new three hundred pounds. Two decades ago William "The Refrigerator" Perry was considered a behemoth in the mid-three hundreds and less than a half dozen players topped three hundred. Today, about 340 NFL players weigh more than three hundred pounds, and there is even one quarterback in that range. It makes for an amazing spectacle. We've perfected the gladiator show, almost eliminating the chance of death. If Heracles were alive today he'd probably make the league, but at his size he'd probably be a linebacker.

But the human body is not something that ought to reflect fashion. It has a proper, perfect, timeless form that reflects strength, balance, agility, and beauty. A man must have muscles, but these should be acquired through heredity and conditioning, not steroids and human growth hormone. The Greek gods still look pretty good 2,500 years later. That look was good enough for my old man, and it's good enough for me. The gods knew what they were doing, and the bronze Zeus or Poseidon in the National Archaeological Museum in Athens certainly has a great build, neither too scrawny nor too buff. I mean, sometimes Greek statuary seems rather modest in penis size, but maybe it was a cold day up there on Mount Olympus.

ON SWIMWEAR

You can tell a lot about a man and what he thinks about himself from his bathing suit. It tells you if he is able to actually and accurately see himself in a mirror. It tells you if he is bold or shy. It may also provide hints as to his social aspirations and/or erotic proclivities.

Is he a guido in a Speedo or a surfer in baggies? Is he strutting his stud stuff in one of those Eurotrash banana hammocks or is he facedown on the beach in a bum-bronzing thong? Or is he impeccably contained in a suit neither too small nor too large, a suit of ambiguous vintage without an apparent sell-by date?

I believe the perfect bathing suit is moderate, modest, and timeless. It is not ironic or humorous. It is not campy like a Hawaiian shirt. It doesn't show off. It doesn't stand out in a crowd. It is decorous in a manly kind of way.

A good bathing suit can compensate for or distract from our physical shortcomings. I want to find the kind of bathing suit that Orson Welles was wearing when he dated Rita Hayworth. I want to find the kind of bathing suit that Mickey Rooney wore on his honeymoon with Ava Gardner. I want to find the kind of bathing suit that Ian Fleming was wearing when he got the seat cushion on his writing chair damp. I want to find a bathing suit like the one Ari was wearing while Jackie lay naked beside him on the sand as frogmen paparazzi stalked the coast. I want to find those Jantzen trunks that Grace Kelly might have yanked off Prince Rainier and thrown, still wet, on a priceless Louis XVI chair. I want those almost Bermuda-length trunks Bobby Kennedy played touch football in on the sand in Acapulco. I want a miracle suit: manly, flattering, confident, beyond reproach.

I want a stoned soul bathing suit. I want a bathing suit that reminds vixens of the song "Don't Mess With 'Mr. T'" by Marvin Gaye. I want a

Rat Pack bathing suit, the kind Frank wore at Twin Palms or Peter Lawford wore when chatting up a little hey-hey with the ring-a-ding chicks at the Tropicana pool. Maybe even an orange one.

I want a bathing suit with at least one and preferably two pockets, or better yet three, one being a small, fold-over interior pocket, a regular feature on many vintage men's suits, a cache for a locker key or a few C-notes.

I want a bathing suit that discreetly complements the man basket yet doesn't reveal whether or not the wearer is circumcised. One of the most significant cultural changes of the "sexual revolution" was the abandonment of the under-suit jockstrap in favor of swinging with abandon, a subtle but important step in the pursuit of freedom. Now we dress for swimming right or left, not just front and center.

I want a bathing suit that doesn't cut into my love handles. I want a suit that makes me a bathing beauty, even if only in the imagination of the beholder. I want a bathing suit that is art.

I want a bathing suit that has neutral buoyancy and never shows ball. I want bathing suits that spruce up the beach; I think some men should wear suits with tops, especially those with a theoretical cup size.

The suave swimmer needs a proper cover-up. I don't expect seaside diners to view my possibly marinara-splashed breasts in a restaurant. A gentleman travels to and from the beach covered. This is where batik sarongs, lavalavas, pareos, African *kikoys,* and other third-worldly accessories belong. After a man unwraps, that decorative fabric can serve as a beach blanket or a pillow, and after a dip, it helps protect the leather seats in the DB5.

The coordinated top-bottom thing—the cabana set—is one great men's mode that never really came back from an unfortunate fashion exile. Men looked great in their matching madras or batik shirts and trunks—the perfect things for poolside lunches. And the once universal terry cloth is tragically underused in après-bathing attire today. A man has to have coverage to and from *la plage* and for the beachside bistro. The sarong is an excellent beach accessory, and it always looks best on globe-trotting heliolaters who bought their sarongs in faraway places with strange-sounding names.

A man needs several bathing suits—enough so that one is always dry. The serious bather also needs bathing shoes. Some of you may scoff, but veterans of the Mediterranean know that it's not all sand out there. There are rocks, medusas, rusty nails, and unharvested *uni*, all waiting to trap the tender foot.

TO BE OR NOT TO BE
IN FASHION

The revolution is coming. I realized this last year, while sitting in the Park Avenue Armory waiting for the Thom Browne men's fashion show to start. I had been reading about gridlock in Congress in the *New York Times* when it suddenly struck me, like a Zeus-bolt from Mount Olympus (2,917 meters), that if we could manage to seriously change men's clothes, the world might change significantly as a consequence. And as the show began and I was looking at a collection that featured men with gauze skirts over their trousers and wearing babushkas and pillbox hats, it somehow seemed to have a sort of magical relationship with the gridlock in Congress, the financial crisis, perhaps even global warming. But let me back up a bit.

Most men think fashion is for women. They think that a man, if he distinguishes himself by his look, is pursuing style, not fashion. Fashion is a group thing. It's what everyone is doing, usually at the behest of a strange, invisible establishment that determines what's in and what's out. Fashion works in mysterious ways, and trends appear simultaneously around the world, as if willed by some superficial god. Fashion doesn't seem to be invented by individual designers as much as it comes out of a collective consciousness or unconsciousness. If men notice it at all, they are likely to ignore it.

I believe that I had convinced myself that men would never participate in fashion in the way women do and that this was, in fact, a good thing. I even had a saying, "I used to be in fashion, but I made bail," which I once thought was a poem. It's not even a good aphorism, and it made my wife frown when I said it. I think she, an unrepentant participant in fashion, thought that this was an insincere statement and that I am far more involved in fashion than I would care to admit. I admit it.

I always loved clothes and I was interested in fashion even as a kid—not just what I wore, but what everyone wore. I think I had a full instinctive understanding of Thorstein Veblen's *Theory of the Leisure Class*, which of course I had never read in elementary school, and aside from the occasions on which I might dress like a cowboy or Tarzan, I happily wore what I thought was in fashion. By the time I reached adolescence, I thought the girls in *Vogue* and *Harper's Bazaar* were infinitely sexier and more interesting than the girls in *Playboy*—distinguishing mammalian attributes being neither very exclusive, nor in the end very stimulating—and the idea of the girl next door didn't appeal to me at all. I lived in Cleveland, Ohio, for one thing. And from there the grand world of *Vogue's* "People Are Talking About" was a fascinating and wonderfully desirable escape. The fashion world seemed to offer a sanctuary from the tedium of the ordinary, and I wanted to go there. And when the miniskirt and Mod-ness happened, fashion's possibilities suddenly seemed genuinely inspiring and relevant. It was like fashion now had a nuclear option—it would end the world as we had known it and take us into a better future, far from home.

Eventually I found myself inside the fashion world, even if I persisted in denying my place in it. I might attend fashion shows and know in considerable detail what was going on, but I could always say that I don't follow the fashions personally. Much. Actually, I felt as if I had a kind of diplomatic immunity to it and that I could dip my toe in when I liked, but when I didn't I had the option of chuckling in refusal. And this remains a tempting posture.

Men's clothes change slowly. My London tailor, Anderson and Sheppard, dates garments on the label, and my suits from '95 and '96 look good today. Some of my favorite ties were bought more than thirty years ago when Calvin Curtis Cravatier went out of business. Not only are they beautiful designs but they're also the perfect width and of beautiful silk that doesn't need a structural foundation. Hey, I have some shirts older than my wife. Men's fashion has long moved at glacier speed. But then once in a while, there's a revolution. And although I am mostly content with how I look, maybe it's time for men to put on some war paint and feathers.

When designers attempt to reinvent menswear, it's hard to pull off. *GQ* has an occasional department called "What Were We Thinking?" which shows big fashion ideas over the years that never caught on, or if they did, that now boggle the mind. What were we thinking in the leisure-suit years of the seventies? Sure they look good on Johnny Depp and Paul Reubens in *Blow*, but if you look at Tony Randall in *The Odd Couple* or Don Knotts in *Three's Company*, you realize that men were experiencing a collective delusion. And today, a decade into the twenty-first century, men's fashion has taken a retro turn, returning us to the vicinity of 1960. Look at *Mad Men* or Tom Ford's *A Single Man*. There's a yen for innocent modernism.

Basically the only difference between men's fashion today and that of a half century ago is the rise of the trousers. Of course, midcentury modern now rules in furniture and architecture as well. Does that mean we realize we've peaked and it's all the same from now on? I wouldn't so much mind staying in 1960 aesthetically, but somehow you know that if you go that route you'll wind up in 1968. The world has moved on too far, and maybe we need a big change in mass fashion just to make history get on with it.

Men's clothes don't change much, but then they do change radically at certain moments in history. Once in a blue moon there's a sartorial sea change, when brave men significantly alter the mode and it actually means something socially and politically. Take Beau Brummell, who was, two hundred years ago, the most famous man in London. Brummell is known as a dandy today, but he was no flaming poof. Au Contraire! What he actually did was turn fashion away from the foppery and the baroque extravagance of the hereditary gentry—eschewing gilt and gaud and wigs—and adopt a relatively sober and restrained costume consisting of a white cravat (his own invention), somber-colored perfectly tailored jackets, and trousers (another innovation of his).

Brummell's style was subtle and urbane, with a sleek, taut cut that favored an athletic body. He declared that if people turn to look at you on the street, you are not well dressed. And this primal manifestation of modernity made him, arguably, the first celebrity: a man famous not for a title (he had none) nor for wealth (his was modest) but for the sheer force of his appearance and personality.

Brummell's eventual downfall occurred when he fell out with his former intimate, George, the Prince of Wales. Speaking to a mutual friend in the presence of the Prince, he quipped, "Who is your fat friend?" Cutting the prince with a quip was, in a way, a more revolutionary act than shooting at him would have been. Brummell's insolence, though with tragic results for himself, indicated that the world had changed forever. A commoner could master a king.

So the age of landed gentry gave way to the age of mercantile democracy, and man, once as florid as a peacock, became as plain as a pigeon. Brummell's costume expressed sobriety, restraint, and common sense (although he himself tended to lack these qualities). And although there was still a class system in play, it would henceforth be a mercantile system divided into white collar and blue collar, management and labor.

But the world turns, and after two centuries of suits and sartorial restraint we've seen rumblings of revolution again. In the last few decades dress codes have quietly vanished from restaurants. Then came Casual Fridays, and when that was accepted, the casual workplace came in and suddenly many jobs that were always performed in suit and tie went all casual all the time. There was mass bafflement. Suddenly the distinction between white collar and blue collar was being blurred or erased. Where it had once been easy to distinguish between rich and poor by their attire, it now became subtle and codified. To tell the difference you had to be able to pick out the $500 dollar jeans. On the surface the casualization of society seemed some sort of a great leveling, a democratic triumph, a visual acknowledgment that we are all one. In fact it was the opposite, since the rich were getting far richer than ever. The lowering of standards of dress simply made it easier for the hyper-rich to hide among us. The guys riding in their Gulfstreams are more likely wearing limited-edition Nike sneakers and Evisu jeans than a Hunstman or Zegna suit. Bill Gates looks like a high school principal. Steve Jobs looks like the gardener. Today a man who is impeccably turned out is probably a haberdasher.

There are, of course, the men we call "suits." These are fellows who wear the business uniform because it's still a part of their profession. They're often middle management, but among the most connected to this traditional cookie-cutter style are politicians, although they tend not to wear good suits. They don't want to look rich, just proper and official, and so they wear baggy suits they don't even think about, and it shows with their trousers bunched up around their shoes and jacket sleeves grazing their knuckles, producing an orangutan-like effect. They wear white buttondowns that they think are dress shirts and loafers that they think are dress shoes. They wear the suit because it is the uniform of capitalist democracy. Those super-capitalists, the Chinese communists, are similarly devoted to the ill-fitting business suit. And when you think about it, it's mostly the suits among us that are holding business and government on traditional, institutional courses ranging from stupid to suicidal.

It's OK to wear the traditional suit and tie if you have great style—that is, if you know how to put the traditional gent's kit together in an original, detailed, almost narrative way. A man can show extraordinary style without really departing from the agreed-upon playing field. But for most men the suit is simply a device that lends them anonymity and immunity from responsibility for their appearance.

There are good reasons for playing the game this way, because there will be consequences if we get involved in fashion hook, line, and sinker like the ladies. Women's fashion is based not only on the idea of social advancement through conspicuous consumption but also on the enforced obsolescence inherent in fashion. Fashion is conspicuous waste. We must be rich because we can toss out our clothes long before they wear out. The fashion person is in a continual reconstruction of his personality because he is defined by a shifting set of symbolic garments.

Fashion is based on the idea of progress, into which we seem to have been bamboozled by science and modernist art. Fashion people say "Oh, that's so last season." And fashion is always a struggle to be up to the moment, if not a millisecond ahead of it. Fashion is based on the idea of forced progress. But unlike science, fashion's progress is not real. We don't dress differently today than we did yesterday because we know more or have learned anything at all. It's novelty for its own sake.

Wyndham Lewis, in *Time and Western Man* (1927): "In the world of Advertisement…everything that happens today (or everything that is being advertised here and now) is better, bigger, brighter, more astonishing than anything that has ever existed before."

If we believed in conspiracies, and we like a good one now and then, we could almost believe that fashion was dreamed up to distract people from more substantial things like government, economics, and social justice. Fashion is more than a huge industry; it has become fully realized as a form of entertainment, a social pathway, indeed it is a profane religion. Fashion is about impalpable beliefs. It is about divining the moment, knowing what everyone will wear and wearing it first, or at least earlier than anyone you know, and then discarding it first to take up the next mode. Fashion is competitive group-think, not individuality. Fashion is not the fingerprint or the snowflake; it is the mold into which the molten fashionables toss themselves to be remade.

And so while it makes sense that serious men do not trifle with fashion, when a sea change arrives—when the paradigm shift hits the fan—it may be that a man has to make his move and go with the inevitable flow of history. We have to understand and accept the ground rules of a revolution. Some men can't tell the difference between a widespread delusion and a sea change. Among better-known delusions of contemporary history: the leisure suit, the power suit, the dickey, platform shoes, lobster-bib ties, and four-or-more-button single-breasted suits. A sea change would describe the recent shift from oversize suit jackets and blousy pleated pants to a trim cut and flat fronts. Just as "if there were no God, it would be necessary to invent him," if there were a classless society, people would have to make some classes up. And so they have. And by their fashions we shall know them.

We now need to go beyond Veblen's conspicuous consumption and conspicuous waste to a theory of conspicuous rebellion. And in the same way that long fingernails and high heels signaled that a person didn't have to perform manual labor, today's extremist fashions announce that the wearer doesn't need to conform or answer to anyone. I can spot a freelancer across a crowded room, the same way I can spot a salesman. A person who can get away with fashion is independent in a way that the compulsory suit wearer or the casual, comfortable dude is not.

If fashion is useful to you, use it. Just don't let it use you. (And it will try.) Fashion is not uninteresting. It's very interesting in its twists and turns. It's tricky. It's not evil, but it's not good either. Nietzsche would probably say that the new Prada collection is "*beyond* beyond good and evil." I won't say "Just say no to fashion." But I might say "Know when to turn the other cheek."

Maybe it's time again for a revolution based on menswear. We need another Brummell. The old order must go. Not just the order of the bad suit, but everything that uniform stands for. Democracies today are paralyzed by corrupt, shortsighted, and self-serving legislatures, agencies, and bureaucracies that toady to the rich in the name of populism. By destroying them stylistically and literally making them look bad, we can usher in a new order. It's not really a new idea. There was the Jacobin liberty cap, the Mao jacket, and Fidel fatigues, but these won't work for us now. We need something new that will clearly separate us from the entropic squares.

Thom Browne's fall 2010 show, the one that made me think that in the next revolution it would be dandies at the barricades of the boardrooms, was held in the grand Tiffany Room at the Seventh Regiment Armory in New York. The Seventh Regiment of the National Guard was the first unit to answer Abraham Lincoln's call for troops at the outset of the Civil War, and somehow it struck me that Browne's radical aesthetic—men in skirts, dresses, babushkas, shorts, and radical revisions of men's tailoring—looked somehow right in an armory. It was a brave display. Of course, designers have been making radical clothing for men for decades now, so how do we know this isn't more stunt stuff to be sold to the rather limited population of window designers and hairdressers eager to sport the latest nutty thing, just like the ladies? Because Browne has already changed the landscape and it looks like we won't be going back. The suits that looked just right a few years back are now looking oddly old; the old jackets are too long, and the old trousers are too long and baggy. There is change in the air.

With Obama's attempts at progressive government hopelessly quagmired by a filibustering conspiracy of plutocratic populists, we need new and unexpected forms of rebellion. If we are to survive with a livable economy and a nontoxic environment, we need to ditch a corrupt, outdated mode of government by which a rabble-rousing media leads the mob against its own interests. Democracy and idiocy are incompatible on one level, de rigueur on another. And so men have to create a revolutionary new identity—one that flaunts intelligence and aestheticism and rejects jive, bourgeois standards. We need an army of individualists determined to stomp out generic personality homogenization and blind party unity.

In the sixties, we rebelled against war by growing long hair and taking to tribal dress, but we can't go back there. This isn't a sit-in. We need a visible rebellion of men who go to work and bring home the uncured, free-range bacon. We need new suits that the corporate suits won't look good in.

Take a look at Washington, Jefferson, and Jackson, and what do you see? Dandies in britches! Beau Brummells with swords and muskets! Men who were unafraid to show off their legs on horseback. Look at Napoleon, and what do you see? A fashion designer with an army! The drab folksy fascists who bamboozle America from the Fox Network and various other organs of befuddlement—and the double-speaking clods in Congress—are cowardly, tasteless, fearful, overweight conformists, hiding in plain sight. They represent by default a cowering public that has given up freedom in fear that their flight to Omaha will hit the jihad lottery and that the president is a deep-cover Muslim. They are ruled by fear at every turn. How quickly might they be banished by hordes of dangerous-looking young rogues, each different from the next, dressed like the hooligans, barbarians, and perverts of their nightmares.

We need a revolution of men in kilts, motorcycle jackets, and down-filled wedding dresses. We need an army of skateboarders in clashing tartans. We need shock troops in berets and goatees, full beards and eyeliner. We need flower-shirted, Roman sandal–wearing bohos, shouting down conservative claptrap with stanzas of beat poetry! We need dreadful dreadlocks in Black Panther leather jackets and gaucho pants setting up guillotines on Wall Street. We need men in top hats and sleek cutaway coats, wielding ivory-handled sword canes they aren't afraid to use against dingy politicians in cheap, ill-fitting suits. If you resemble the masses, you are the enemy. If your appearance is complex, evocative, and unique as a snowflake, welcome to the avalanche of individuality that will bury the totalitarian drones of the status quo!

Don't give up your style, men, but don't ignore how the handwriting on the wall is fashioned. The world is turning beneath our feet.

GETTING IT PERFECTLY WRONG

"Nothing is true, everything is permitted."

—Hassan-i Sabbah

"No shoes, no shirt, no service."

—Proverb

Rules? There are no stinking rules. It's all what you can get away with. Every moment of every day the world turns and, voilà, revolution! People believe that there are rules of dressing because someone told them—probably their grandma. Of course, there are rules that some people live by, because of the general dearth of common sense, sense of occasion, and the scarcity of savoir faire. And that's OK. Most guys have no eye, no ear, no knowledge, and no feel. Grandmas are correct in telling you the rules as they have learned them, about when to wear white and what to wear at night. This is because grandmas have common sense and they think you don't. But if you know the rules and you have both common sense and your own style, you can do as you please and pull it off. The rules are all out the window anyway because it's the end of the world; at least, it is in the movies.

Once you get your look perfect, it's time to fuck it up. Add some charming defects, mannerisms, and discrepancies. If you look at photos of the dashing majordomo of early twentieth-century bohemia, Ezra Pound, his dandy look often features one shirt collar up and one shirt collar down. This is one of my personal favorite affectations, Ezra-ing the chemise.

One collar should be in its usual place, the other askew. A variant is one buttondown buttoned, one flying free.

Who wants to look impeccable, i.e., perfectly conforming to a real or imagined standard, when you can be fascinatingly peccable? You don't want to look too innocent, mild mannered, or uptight. If there is nothing wrong with your look, you don't look right.

The tie is a prime location for deviant self-expression. A knot should almost always be asymmetrical. I like a tie that looks like it was tied without looking. Another tactic is to allow the tip of the narrow end of the tie to hang below the tip of the wide end. This is a favorite trick of Italian dandies, but it can be overdone. I once met with the chairman of a major publishing house, and the spectacular dominance of the narrow end alone made me suspect he had returned from a multi-martini lunch. Salvador Dalí believed that if one tie was good, two were even better.

The pocket hankie presents almost infinite possibilities for eccentricity. Linen or silk hanging way out of the jacket pocket is in common usage, but it tends to be show-offish and the sign of a loud talker or narcissistic lout. The hankie has a language of its own. I say "hankie" because hopefully the "pocket square" will be abandoned as the mark of a square. The white handkerchief, or colored variants in cotton or linen, both launderable fabrics, is infinitely preferable to a colored piece of silk with no utility. (And a matching pocket square and tie is simply out of the question.) Why the hankie and not the silk square? Well, you can blow your nose on it. Or give it to your sobbing wife, or use it as a tourniquet or to stop up a bullet hole. The TV fold, popular in the fifties, is in again, showing a neat white rectangle over the breast pocket. The pointed fold, in which the corners of the hankie show above the pocket, is also worn now. Some men take care that the little triangles form a neat line above the pocket, like sailboats in a regatta, while others simply hold the hankie in the middle and jam it into the pocket, letting the corners pop up in a more organically floral way. It's a matter of which way your wind blows. There's the puff, in which none of the corners are visible, the hankie rising out of the pocket like a cloud. Then there is the triangle, which is more or less the TV fold on an angle. Some men use one of these approaches; some men use several or all of them, depending on their mood. I like all of these techniques, depending on the jacket I'm wearing or how I'm feeling.

Untied shoes were once outside the realm of possibility for a gent, but now it seems that it's the next step after socklessness. We see the untied Adidas look popularized by Run DMC employed by Berluti-wearing dandies. My natty, bespoke-suited friend Wayne Maser can be found sockless with laces flying loose in all seasons. Somehow he manages not to step on the laces and fall. I guess keeping them short is important. The lace-less look, like pants on the ground, can probably be traced back to the jail-house, where shoelaces are confiscated so they can't be used for suicide by hanging. How anyone could hang themselves with their shoelaces, I've never understood. Maybe with those rawhide Timberland-style laces. But what it says is "I'm self-employed" or "I don't care" or "Don't tread on me."

Another Wayne tactic: under his crisp, white shirt he doesn't wear a T-shirt but a tight Henley, and his French cuffs are not closed with cufflinks but gold twist ties from cookie bags of a certain fancy bakery. The great ones are innovators. I've always hated white T-shirts visible under an open collar, but during the heyday of the GAP pocket tee I liked combining colored T-shirts with colored shirts—giving a sort of casual Ascot effect.

Fred Pressman, the late chairman of Barneys New York, was one of the most elegant and stylish men I have known. Fred's suits were works of art. They were all bespoke, made by Kiton and other tailors, and his shoes were handmade. But Fred liked to wear shirts frayed at the collar and cuffs—particularly his custom-made buttondowns—adding an element of "so what?" to an otherwise flawless appearance. I even suspected Fred's occasional displays of dandruff to be deliberate.

Black and brown is supposed to be a bad combination. Vincent Gallo makes it look good. I was always told as a kid that both blue and black and blue and green are bad combinations, when in fact they can be among the best. The potter Jonathan Adler's manifesto says "We believe colors can't clash." I don't think they can either, unless they really want to.

A hint of cross-dressing always gets attention. It didn't hurt Nirvana's band members' careers to wear housedresses in a video, because they were so obviously non-drag types. Kurt Cobain's style utilized a lot of appropriated femininity and it just made him more of a hetero sex symbol—like the floral yoked sweaters he wore. I wore the same kind of girl cardigans when I was his age and weight without any misinterpretation. I think Keith Richards was the instigator of the butch androgyny thing. In his autobiography, he writes about picking up his girlfriend Anita's clothes because they were the same size. I don't borrow much from my wife, but I will swipe the occasional scarf or borrow her sunglasses.

Like most men, I have always had an affection for worn-out clothes. When I first moved to New York and began hanging out at Max's Kansas City I was wearing my preppy clothes from college days, some of them quite shredded. I remember arguing with punk sex symbol Richard Hell over who had started the fashion for wearing ripped clothes. We both felt responsible. Today's youths have a similar taste for wear and tear, but they don't have the perspicacity to achieve the state of artfully disheveled without assistance. Hence there is a vast industry involved in the mass production of faded, abraded, ripped, torn, and stained clothes, particularly jeans. We've been through acid-washed and stonewashed. I consider distressed clothing the height of decadence. I was sent a free pair of a replica of the oldest-known extant pair of Levi's. They are cool looking and comfortable and they have braces buttons and the buckled belt in the back that I like but I just can't bring myself to wear them. Women get upset if they run into a woman wearing the same dress, and I find the idea of running into someone wearing pants with exactly the same rips and stains actually creepy.

When it comes to deliberate departures, it is important to abandon them as soon as they get too popular. When polo shirts became the fashion a large segment of the polo-istas began flipping the collars up. A gentleman who belonged to the same golf club I did was in the habit of wearing the collars of his Ralph Lauren polo shirts up. I didn't mind these shirts, because his initials are also R.L. I thought they worked better on him than usual. But as we were regular golf partners, the collar up began to grate on me, so I adopted a simple but effective technique. Every time he came out of the locker room I would say, "Hey Bobby, your collar is up in the back." Within one season I wore him and his collar down.

Some gestures are just too much. The first time I met David Bowie he was wearing an interesting outfit with outsize pants and Mary Jane pumps—and it was all working, except for the two different-colored socks. That looked like he was trying too hard. I think one was red and one was bright blue. Now, if one was black and one was dark gray that would have been interesting. But a year later he was Ziggy Stardust and beyond sartorial good and evil.

Time warp is always good, throwing something in the mix from another decade, century, or millennium like jewelry, a scarf, or an ancient tie. Fred Astaire used ties as belts, a good trick for the slim of figure. Ethnic items can function like spice in an outfit. My friend Hooman, who is basically a very stylish Savile Row man, wears traditional Persian cotton shoes that he has dyed green in support of the new Iranian revolution. Stefano Pilati has taken up those South Asian pants that look like the ones MC Hammer wore. *Vogue*'s European editor Hamish Bowles wears colored slipperlike shoes, and his bespoke suits seem to suggest that his fabric searches sometimes take him beyond the suitings department into the upholstery and drapery section, but to very good effect. Boutonnieres are always unexpected these days, and rare flowers can transport one's look. Why not put a four-leaf clover in your buttonhole? Or a sprig of mistletoe around the holidays? Or some small maple leaves you can claim are poison ivy? When it comes to getting dressed, well enough should never be left alone.

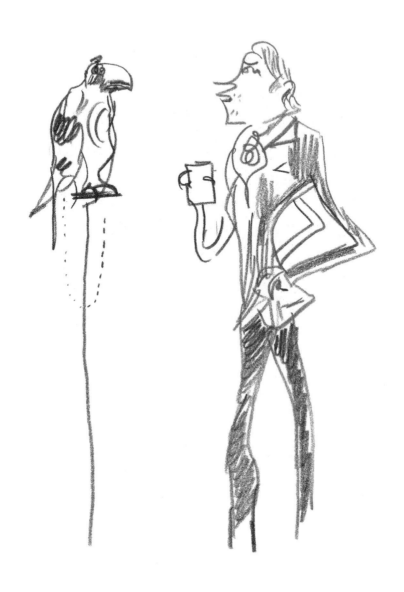

HOW TO COMMUNICATE

The Human Voice

Our personal instrument can be a source of eloquence and poetry, or it can be a noisome noise tantamount to pollution of the civil environment. We must guard not only our words but also our tone. How often have we encountered a fellow with an "outdoor voice" and wished he had a volume-control knob? Talking too loudly is a basic offense, like standing too closely: it violates the physical conventions of human interaction. Of course, the loud talker is probably unaware of his offense, and it may actually result from his being hard of hearing, but as often as not it results from a bombastic temperament given to boast and bluster.

There is no reason to put up with loud louts. I suggest that when such a broadcast is aimed at one's face, the appropriate response is to move the shoulders and head back quickly, as if dodging a punch. Repeat this maneuver as needed. Or try the rejoinder "I hear you." Or nod knowingly and distinctly declare, "Say no more!"

Almost as irritating as the outdoor talker is the low talker—the person whose words are barely audible. (A famous episode of *Seinfeld* addresses this problem.) The only appropriate response is to let the low talker know that you cannot hear what he or she is saying. "I beg your pardon" or "Sorry" will probably not suffice. I suggest getting it over with once and for all by saying, "Excuse me, but I cannot hear a word you are saying." If you like, you can soften it a bit by adding that in your youth you played in a thrash metal band or served in the artillery and may be a tad deaf, but save yourself repeated interjections and possible misunderstandings by making it clear that you are not receiving.

And you: By all means, speak up! Moderately, clearly, and distinctly. Say what you mean, mean what you say, and say it like you mean it.

Telephonery: The Landline

Most of us still have a telephone connected to the network by wires. The so-called landline, often declared obsolete, is a good alternative to a mobile because you can hire someone to answer it or you can have it answered by machine. The landline gives you a number at which you may be unreachable. I have cordless phones in my home and office, but I prefer a phone with a cord. It makes me feel grounded and secure, sure that no one is listening in from the next building and that I am reducing the electronic traffic through my skull. Am I paranoid? Perhaps, but I think it's more of an affectation I picked up from the *Battlestar Galactica* series, in which phones with cords were used to provide greater security from the inhuman cybernetic race, the Cylons.

If you can afford it, hire a person with a BBC accent to answer your telephone. If you must pick up your own phone, answer it "Hello, studio." In New York City, many landlines are answered "Hello, studio," or simply "Studio." This is a glamorous way to answer, suggesting that you have reached an art studio or a photo studio—possibly even a movie studio or massage parlor. It is an especially good way to answer the phone when the call has awakened you, as the caller may be temporarily confused, giving you a moment to achieve full wakefulness and realize where you are.

I recommend having at least two lines so that if you want to get off a call, you can dial your landline from your mobile phone and your second line will ring audibly, giving you an out. It is also more professional than a call-waiting beep, as it conjures up a busy workplace.

If you are called by someone you dislike or someone you don't know—perhaps someone attempting to collect a debt—inquire who is calling, then add "May I ask what this is about?" after which you may put them on punitive hold and neglect to return to the line.

When you receive sales calls or solicitations on your home phone, you can try retaliating by sounding a marine air horn into the receiver, but use discretion as these can be heard a mile away. A more discreet approach is to ask the callers for their home number so that you can return the call in the evening. ("Oh, you don't like being called at home?") A classic revenge on telemarketers is to answer the phone, pretend that you are a detective on a murder scene, and begin to interrogate the caller, asking what business he had with the victim.

When you have a cold, or when visitors who are possibly contagious use your phone, sterilize it after use. If you have an answering machine, when recording your message resist the temptation to play DJ and provide a musical interlude or try out your stand-up comedy routine. People like me will hate you for wasting seconds of their time. Never say "You have reached [your name here]." Obviously the caller will be talking to a machine because he has not reached [your name here], and when he does, it will be in the future. If you must say your name, say "Eventually you will have reached [your name here]." Or simply repeat your number and add, "Please leave a message." This will inform any wrong numbers that they have erred without revealing your identity, which is likely to be more fabulous than theirs, tempting them to stalk you in the future.

If a form you are filling out requires a telephone number, give your fax. The fax machine, incidentally, should be located as far away from your bed as possible in the event of incoming nocturnal Japanese business.

Telephonery: The Mobile

Mobile phones are like the Wizard of Oz: great and terrible. They make us more efficient. We are now reachable most of the time and have no need for pockets full of filthy quarters. Theoretically, we can accomplish more work. But at what cost? How good is it to be constantly reachable? We realize when we create fictional automotive viaducts—lying through our teeth with a "Sorry, I'm going into a tunnel"—that there are times we want radio silence, unavailability, and a Garbo-like aloneness. And then there are those moments of clarity when one realizes that those Bluetooth-eared businessmen walking on Park Avenue talking to themselves are in a real sense actually talking to themselves. You can tell by the vacant gaze and lumbering gait that they have essentially beamed up to Planet Cubicle. Not a pretty sight.

Do not become one of them. Do not be a phone drone. Do not walk the streets talking into a digital parasite. Find a bench or duck into an entranceway, lest you become another roaming zombie clogging our sidewalks with inattention and stepping in front of speeding taxicabs.

There are places for the mobile in modern society. A restaurant is not one of them. Upon entering a restaurant, a gentleman silences his phone. Allowing one's phone to ring in a restaurant or theater is an offense deserving of shunning or ostracism (in the classical sense—no one should give you food, water, or fire). It is generally rude to answer one's mobile phone at the table unless absolutely vital information is expected, preferably pertaining to both you and your companion, such as an expected date being lost in an avalanche.

To answer a mobile phone during sex should be grounds for divorce and a mitigating factor in homicide charges. Other forbidden zones for mobile phones are elevators, places of worship, funeral homes, poetry readings, trains, airplanes, museums, art galleries, theaters, waiting rooms, gyms, yoga studios, and concerts.

Anywhere their use would annoy or distract others is off-limits for mobile phones. Audience members should refrain from phoning except in places where their use is virtually impossible anyway because of background noise, like stadiums and sports arenas. I attended the funeral of a good friend once, and despite an announcement beforehand, the service was painfully interrupted several times by ringing phones. In today's world of hip-hop ringtones, such rude oversights can lead to grotesque situations. And don't think the vibrate setting exempts you. It's more than a pin drop during Hamlet's soliloquy.

Still, the overarching problem with mobile phones is not *where* they are used but *how*. We accept actual person-to-person conversations next to us in public places; it's the cellular field holler/hog-call loudness of speech that is infuriating. If people in your vicinity can listen to your end of the conversation, you are speaking too loudly. Often the disembodying effect of the mobile phone deprives insensitive persons of any appropriate sense of place, bringing into a public arena intimate subject matter we would rather not share in—windfall profits, why she left him, his powerlessness over alcohol, urinary tract infections. We don't want to know the lurid details of strange lives. These should stay where they belong, behind closed—and locked—doors.

Theoretically, the texting and e-mail features of today's phones are more socially acceptable than the speech mode, but not if someone is pecking away with his pinkie while the two of you are in conversation. Texters and typers should excuse themselves from the presence of others and go do their tiny typing in the toilet. Recently I found myself announcing loudly to a texter at an ATM, "It's not a phone booth!"

The mobile phone ring itself is a pernicious annoyance. The vibrate feature communicates to the phone's owner only and is therefore the preferred option in most instances. Long melodic passages and electronica of the sort one might hear on television dramas where electronically fused explosives are counting down are also annoying in the extreme. The old-school telephone ring simulating an actual bell once seemed refreshing, but today so many mobile users have that ring that it's common to see an entire room reach into its pockets at the first trill. If you must have an audible ringtone, select the least offensive one possible. You are what you beep.

Warning Shots

When one encounters flagrant cellular-etiquette violators and a glare doesn't do it, some good old-fashioned throat clearing can be an effective and enjoyable play. If the offender's thickness is not easily penetrable, you can quote Ratso Rizzo: "Hey, I'm walking here!" Or try a good paraphrase: "Hey, I'm thinking here," or "Hey, I'm reading here."

Or "Is that a cell phone or a bullhorn?"

On the train or the treadmill, it's sometimes easier just to move away from the wireless primate; you don't want to have to punch it. However, if the offender is in violation of the local ground rules, by all means rat him out. Omertà does not apply to loud phone talkers. If they annoy you, they annoy others. And sometimes a good, loud "I beg your pardon?" delivered in a tone similar to what you might use if the fellow had grabbed your butt, offers the correct dose of righteous indignation.

There will always be emergencies. It's OK to take a call if it involves birth, death, or infinity. But when you are enjoying the company of physically present persons, it's best to turn the mobile off unless you are waiting for your theater tickets or the limo. If it's your first date—and you want a second—you should probably turn the phone off entirely. Lingering outside a restaurant or in the restroom during a date to make phone calls, text, or check voice or e-mail is just as bad an idea as making people wait to empty their bladders while you hoover up blow in the men's room.

E-Mail

Electronic mail lacks the dignity of the traditional variety, but it is not so much the engraved high-rag-content stationery that makes the difference as the state of mind. Letter writers assume that there are rules to be followed while e-mailers simply follow the bad examples of their peers.

Always answer invitations and do so promptly, even annoying party e-vites. Just say no and nip it in the bud. I have found that the best policy is to return every phone call, because in the long run it will save you time and anxiety and give you the reputation of a man who gets things done. If you really don't want to speak to someone, call him back at lunchtime. Leave a message that you are traveling. E-mail if possible. I have always found that truly important and/or famous people get right back to you—it's the pretentious assistants you can't get through to. What's the lesson there?

Sometimes having a carbon footprint seems not all that bad. Spared the cost of paper, printing, and postage, press agents and advertisers clog our mailboxes with impunity. "E-mail blasts" are broadcast to enormous lists at the push of a key. Unprofessional morons neglect to blind carbon copy when sending out a "blast," exposing your e-mail address to hundreds or thousands more potential e-stalkers. With e-mail, etiquette can be counterintuitive; it is often rude to be too polite. When someone replies to you, it is not necessary to thank them, generating a chain reaction of chores.

Then there are obtrusive attachments. How many times, in an e-mail-volume-addled state, have I downloaded a MIME attachment that turned out to be nothing more than a corporate logo or signature? Trust me: attaching a Facebook or Twitter logo to your e-mail will only make me hate you. Attaching a logo to your correspondence is pretentious. The golden rule of e-mail is don't waste the time of others, lest they waste yours. There ought to be a law.

Hopefully, at some time in the future, etiquette and even laws will ensure that time lost is taken seriously. When some dumb driver cracks up on the parkway, causing cars containing 800 people to be delayed for an hour, the human cost is 800 hours. The culprit should pay up in kind, ten workweeks or the equivalent in paychecks! If time is money, let's make it liquid.

Letters

Letter writing is a lost art in more ways than one. When I look at mail from earlier eras, I behold the cursive with melancholy admiration. How beautiful was that collaboration between the mind and the pen! Musicians have told me that my typestroking is quite rhythmic, but that's no substitute for a gorgeous hand.

Putting it down on paper, except when promising or threatening, is such a nice formality. Thank-you notes should be written on stationery whenever possible. Softies like me often save them, convinced by the effort that the senders were truly grateful.

And few things are more charming than a handwritten, postmarked letter. I feel an endangered sort of joy when opening one. The obsolescence of physical correspondence is tragic. I can't envision *The Collected E-mails of Glenn O'Brien*. Well, maybe a Kindle Original.

THE CORRECT INSULT

"When it comes down to pure ornamental cursing, the native American [miner] is gifted above the sons of men."

—Mark Twain, *Buffalo Express*, Dec. 18, 1869

When it comes to choosing our words, precision and accuracy are essential. Misunderstandings caused by inaccurate language frequently create arguments, assaults, murders, suicides, feuds, and divorces, not to mention invasions, blockades, and carpet bombing.

In the ordinary course of communication, we have excellent aids in the pursuit of correct usage. Within reach I have *Fowler's Modern English Usage*, which explains clearly and concisely the difference between "regretful" and "regrettable," "inquire" and "enquire," and a *Dictionary of Contemporary American Usage*, which guides me when I have to decide whether I am constantly, continually, continuously, perpetually, or incessantly angered by the government. ("Constantly" is the choice, since my vexation is interrupted by intervals of sleep.)

I am also armed with several volumes of intelligent discussions of meaning, such as Kingsley Amis's *The King's English*, which brings Fowler up to date, and *Words in Sheep's Clothing*, by Mario Pei, which discusses assaults on meaning from journalists, politicians, bohemians, and other practitioners of rhetoric. While sharpening my weaponry, these tools have also made me even crankier, and I find my goat has been gotten more and more often by folks attempting to be fancy in their language.

We are living through a plague of failed eloquence. I find myself frequently retained to supply "verbiage." If the fee offered is not princely,

I tend to point out to the prospective client that "verbiage" means an abundance of useless words such as one might encounter in legislatures. Is that what they really want? Or do they want some catchy copy? Another peeve regarding the lily gilders is "plethora," which I hear all the time pretending to mean "abundance." "Plethora" means "too much" and is not to be used positively and invitingly. It belongs to the vocabulary of complaint. There is a plethora of "plethora" misusers.

But for all the excellent reference books on language, I find no guide to the correct use of slang, in the use of which precision is no less valuable. I think there's an entire book here, but I would like to get the ball rolling by offering some notes on words we hear every day in America but read far less often.

If you wish to insult a person, vague generalities are ineffective and often counterproductive. It pays to be as precise and specific as possible. Anyone can launch a barrage. It takes skill to be a marksman of aspersion. Here is a brief guide to the correct use of common epithets.

Dick; dickhead; shit: A dick is a careless egotist who abuses others in demonstration of his high and misplaced self-regard. This egocentrist, who might have once been called a cad, is always mean-spirited, self-aggrandizing, and aggressive. A dickhead is similarly uncaring and overconfident but generally with less intelligence and skill. The dickhead's misdeeds are less accomplished than those of the dick. Dick Cheney is a dick; George Bush is a dickhead. A shit is also a person inclined to take pleasure in the misfortune of others, although perhaps less out of self-regard than misanthropy. The shit may be more passively malignant than a dick, unless he is a total shit. It is possible, however, to be both a dick and a shit. Both Bush and Cheney are shits.

"Cocksucker" is a term that has become disconnected from its literal meaning. No doubt its origin is homophobic, but whereas the act of sucking a cock seems subservient and submissive and is likely to be tender, "cocksucker" has come to mean an arrogant, malignant, nasty, and aggressive man. It is the modern equivalent of "knave" verging on "churl." "Cockbiter" would be truer to literal sense, but that's unlikely to catch on.

A similar disconnect has developed recently with the adjective "gay," as in "That's so gay." The original use was homophobic, but the usage may now carry little conscious, deliberate disregard for homosexuals. To some, "gay" means ineffectual, twee, wimpy, or alien. It is used mostly by persons to whom variety and intelligence are alien. Ironically this usage itself is so gay, in the nongay sense of gay.

"Faggot" is used less and less exclusively as a derogatory term for homosexuals and more and more as a term for an unmanly man with little fortitude, i.e., a wimp. In this sense "faggot" may be approaching its original meaning, referring to a bundle of twigs, as the individual so designated is likely to be an insubstantial conformist. Since it still carries an antihomosexual bias, however, anyone who uses "faggot" is a faggot. Except in the case of some gays for whom this F-word functions as the N-word does among blacks: they find offense in its use by others but not by their own.

An asshole is a person with a delusional worldview who is incapable of observing social boundaries. Assholes are rude, uncaring, and ridiculous. The asshole may flout the rules consciously or unconsciously. The asshole exhibits a diminished or deficient superego. He may be a less accomplished sociopath and may also verge on psychotic, in which case he may be termed a flaming asshole. Unfortunately, the sort so referred to slanders one of our most useful and hopefully reliable organs, an organ that is a source of relief, even joy.

An ass is similar to an asshole, but is less vigorous and flamboyant. An ass is a persistent fool, a dullard perhaps. "Asswipe," popularized by *Beavis and Butthead,* is similar to an ass kisser, brownnoser, or arse licker.

"Cunt," a word that is very popular in Britain and which in Australia borders on the affectionate, is extremely inflammatory when applied to women in the United States, and feminists may eventually seek imprisonment for those who use the term. A cunt is a mean-spirited, hairsplitting, vindictive person who enjoys the suffering of others—particularly if he is the cause of that suffering. The cunt is also unsympathetic and tends toward cruelty and schadenfreude. Cunts are black-belt wet blankets often drawn to positions of authority or even law enforcement, although they usually lack courage. A hall monitor is likely to be a cunt; a SWAT team member is not. A cunt is given to one-upsmanship and meddling. A twat lacks the talent, intelligence, or energy to be a true cunt.

A fuckhead is a person of poor judgment but considerable enthusiasm. A fuckhead is generally stupid and persistent in his stupidity. (See "dipshit," below.) A fuck is a person who enjoys unpleasant encounters—"fucking with you" and presenting gratuitous difficulty.

Wanker; jackoff; jerk: All these terms refer to a person involved in actions that are masturbatory in their ineffectuality or fruitlessness. They refer to persons engaged in noticeably unproductive, unintelligent, and generally repetitive behavior. A wanker is always ineffectual, although he may be unaware of his lack of effect, and quite affected. (See "poser.")

Geek; dork; dweeb; nerd; doofus: All these terms refer to persons who exist outside the alpha-male realm and sensibility, eschewing, consciously or not, traditional modes of masculinity. A computer company has a TV advertising campaign based on its employees' pride in being geeks; another refers to its technical consultants as "the geek squad." "Geek" originally referred to carnival employees who bit the heads off chickens, and as practitioners of this trade tended to be outsiders, it came to mean people with little concern for mainstream interests. It is basically synonymous with "nerd," a word apparently derived from Dr. Seuss's *If I Ran the Zoo*. Both "geek" and "nerd" have been reclaimed by those so called, who are proud of the qualities that brought the appellation, much as "queer" has been proudly adopted by its intended targets. "Geek" and "nerd" both convey a certain expertise. However, while the dork has the outsider manners of the geek and the nerd and the same disregard for style, he is without any particular skill or accomplishment, although he may have intelligence without awareness. Likewise, a dweeb is an asocial person without effect, a failed geek or nerd. A doofus is generally a clumsy nerd without the intelligence to make it as a dork or a geek.

Dipshit: a nerdy fuckhead.

Dickbrain: someone whose behavior is not ruled by the frontal lobe but by the lower centers of the brain; i.e., the little head vetoes the better instincts of the big head.

"Motherfucker" is a very powerful word with a broad spectrum of meanings. In the negative and most literal sense, a motherfucker is a person who flouts taboos, without conscience or principles. But more often "motherfucker" indicates seriousness, gravity (or gravitas), and power, as in "a real motherfucker." A motherfucker may be the worst or the best, depending on the situation, but in every case, except as a term of casual affection, it connotes transcendence of the norm.

A douche bag is a loser who may yet exhibit a certain vanity and overconfidence. Despite being widely recognized as deficient or worthless, the douche bag (or "douche") persists in an attitude of self-infatuation. A douche bag is, in short, a narcissist without reason. His lack of talent makes him only an accessory to a cunt.

A bozo is a clown or a fool but with a connotation of active energy or even aggression. He is outlandish, out of touch, and probably ineffectual though highly visible.

Scumbag: a person who delights in the misery of others and who will do his best to contribute to that misery if it is convenient and without onerous repercussions. A scumbag is generally devious and fraudulent, and both meaner and more malevolent than a plain dick.

"Tool" is similar to "fool," but it implies that the person's inane or stupid actions may be in service of something or someone beyond his ken. He may believe that he is getting over on others, while in reality others have gotten over on him. Thus, the Republican Party counts many tools as members. A tool has more delusions of self-possession than a simple fool and he may fancy himself a stud and a hustler.

A prick is a dick but with the connotation of more deliberate and planned malice. A prick is less formidable than a cunt.

Bitch; bastard; son of a bitch: "Bitch" is an umbrella term for a person of ill will manifest through feminine forms. "Bastard" is a catchall term for a person of ill will manifest through masculine forms. In urban usage, "bitch" can be a casual reference to any female not one's own mother; it is also synonymous with a beta male or anyone suspected of or exhibiting submissive behavior. "Bitch" may also be used as a term of admiration, especially in regard to rate of difficulty or tricky forms of power. "Son of a bitch" may be freely substituted for "bastard."

Shithead; shit for brains: an idiot or moron. Someone lacking cognitive and reasoning powers, unlike a shit, who is not without resources.

Pussy is, of course, a highly desirable commodity in the ordinary course of things, but when applied to a man, it means that he is a coward, sissy, or weakling. An empowered pussy is a cunt. "Wuss" may be a euphemism for pussy, or like "wimp" it may indicate a less spectacular brand of cowardice.

"Ho," that lightning-rod word, may yet prove to be the feminist N-word, as it could be turned against those who use it lightly or in a casual hip-hop context. Hos are persons of loose morals who sell themselves without regard for moral standards. In today's world, "ho" can applied to most people. Shock-jock Don Imus was fired by CBS for using the word "ho." If Imus had called the women in question "meretricious" he would have never had a problem.

The above epithets are all useful in their own way, but consider the allure of an insult that not only sounds bad but is also more specific and possibly foreign to the recipient, who may, upon hearing it, feel even more stupid. Confusion over arcane terms of contumely can only help drive the point home to a lickspittle, toady, stumblebum, rube, bounder, middlebrow, mythomaniac, charlatan, yokel, lout, or schmendrick. And those words just feel good on the tongue.

HOW TO FIGHT LIKE A MAN

Testosterone may have *something* to do with it, if one would believe or indulge pop-feminist thinking. Too much testosterone! How many times have we heard that spurious and demeaning explanation of some ugly event? And not just when we are engaged in spontaneous mortal combat or impromptu sportive barroom brawling—even at the slightest display of assertiveness.

It is well known that some of the most vicious fights of all fall into the category of the catfight, aka bitch fight, wherein two women go *womano a womano,* no holds barred, battling tooth and nail out of pure…could it be estrogen?

Luckily, catfighters are generally too vain to do much damage. If they knew what they were doing, the furious assailants might kill each other. Women seem far more pitiless and remorseless than men. Should you witness such a rare but brutal fight break out and you are in the company of the sort of woman who might tend to blame male dustups, road rage, or even global political tensions on too much testosterone, do not lose this valuable opportunity to comment, "Too much estrogen!"

Men fight because they know how. They have been trained or even bred for it. Fighting is natural and often it is simply a way for them to pass the time, particularly if they are not very intelligent and educated. For some human males, it is simply how they discuss things, and for a lot of men, grappling is as close as they can get to hugging and kissing one another. Most men are most comfortable around men, and sometimes striking one another may simply be a way to express mutual admiration. I have noticed this on the streets of Ireland during pub hours. One rarely encounters such behavior in the United States anymore, probably due to the high percentage of attorneys in our population.

Men are brutes and beasts by nature. It's probably residual survival instincts—we've had relatively few centuries in which we weren't threatened by lions, tigers, and bears—oh my!—not to mention tribal war parties. And then there's ritual display of combat prowess for the wooing of eligible "nubiles." In some species, males battle to impress females with their ability to protect them; in other species, males resort to extravagant display of their wares. I recommend ware display as a far more enjoyable form of natural selection, and for many of us, a far more winnable one as well.

The instincts of fight and flight are still hardwired into our bodies. Any reading of the classics will lead you to conclude that we are a race of murderers and that the ability to slaughter is high on the list of traditionally desirable attributes. According to Homer, the accursed rage of Achilles brought pain to thousands, and the hero of Irish myth, Cúchulainn, killed a hundred men per day, so the comparative peace the planet now enjoys could be seen as a remarkable sign of progress.

One function of civilization, therefore, is the moderation of the homicidal instinct, and we manage to do this through strategic sublimation: film and television war dramas, football and hockey, boxing, wrestling, and ultimate fighting, and, of course, video games. (In our house, we ritually slaughter one another in *Call of Duty: Black Ops*.) As a race we have managed to mostly suppress gladiatorial contests to the death, but in sports, shit happens and sometimes someone is crippled with the old helmet-to-helmet spear hit, or maimed or snuffed in a NASCAR rollover; however, are these not better ways to go than in a coughing spasm in an oxygen tent? I have often thought "Live fast, die young, and leave a good-looking corpse" to be good advice. For other people.

A gentleman is a man civilized to the degree that he can channel his homicidal impulses into socially condoned arenas, such as sports, the military, the police, or business. Nevertheless, a gentleman should always be prepared to defend himself should he come under attack from non-gentlemen, gentlemen with whom he does not agree, their agents, or women.

Defense against women is the most difficult of all, since unprovoked hostile attacks by females will often be characterized as self-defense since the woman is widely considered to be the weaker sex. The preemptive strike is an old female stratagem. Obviously women are not really the weaker sex, since they invariably survive their husbands after defeating them in a thousand ways. But since they are often smaller and possess less physical strength, they can easily position themselves as underdogs or victims.

When attacked by a woman or women, unless there is no possibility of escape, the wisest course is flight. You cannot fight back against a woman, even with reliable witnesses who will testify to the defensive nature of your actions, because any injury you might cause your attacker will be seen as evidence of your brutality as long as you live. You can only fend off attack while attempting to escape, after which you can seek an order of protection from the authorities or attempt to have your attacker institutionalized.

When an altercation occurs between gentlemen, they usually find a way to resolve it without resorting to violence, and even when violence is used, traditionally it has been governed by certain principles. Dueling with swords or pistols was once considered the way gentlemen resolved serious grievances. Dueling has even enjoyed periods of great fashionability.

The idea of the duel is combat between two individuals of the supposed gentry with matched weapons and according to certain rules. The duel was fought on what was known as a "field of honor," and presumably it was fought over what was perceived as a slight to one man's honor by the other.

Dueling has been generally illegal since the seventeenth century, although society often looked the other way. In 1804 Alexander Hamilton, the leading Federalist politician and first secretary of the United States Treasury, was killed in a duel by Aaron Burr, the sitting vice president of the United States. Burr was charged with murder, but the charges were dropped.

Today dueling is seriously frowned upon and should anyone suggest a duel, you should immediately notify your attorney and suggest that the challenger do the same. While a man may wish to kill you, he will not want to be billed by the hour to do so.

If we have been raised to be gentlemen, we have probably been taught that gentlemen fight within the rules. This principle may have been the case when combat was common and weapons crude, but observing rules in today's world would be entirely speculative and one would be a fool to voluntarily relinquish advantages. True, many men fight with a certain restraint, considering biting, eye gouging, and blows to the privates to be out of bounds. Women will generally not observe any such niceties in attacks on your person. I suggest that a gentleman should not, either, and that he make every effort to win an unavoidable combat in as short a time as possible.

Consider the cold cock as a way of saving everyone time and blood loss. Cold cock is not a Jamaican appetizer or a winter complaint but a form of combat based on preemption. Assuming that you are the first to realize that violence is imminent and unavoidable, you strike your adversary with sufficient force to induce immediate unconsciousness or, at the very least, an effective stupor upon which you retire from the field with dignified haste.

My number one rule of fighting has nothing to do with the Marquess of Queensberry—that most famous rule maker for fisticuffs was also the vindictive fellow who persecuted Oscar Wilde and saw him sent to jail, and who among us ought to observe anything he deemed proper? Instead, consider the practicality of the situation. It is imperative to win a fight in the first five or ten seconds. The older one gets, the more important this rule becomes. And winning doesn't mean injuring your opponent; it simply means disabling, disorienting, or indisposing him in order to prevent further escalation and possible injury to either party. Bloody noses and hallucinated stars have prevented many serious injuries.

I haven't been in a fight in years, and if I got in one I might have a heart attack (if I didn't win in the first ten seconds), but I have been in numerous fights in my lifetime. The last one, as far as I recall, was at a loft party in the latter part of the twentieth century, when I became involved in grappling and fisticuffs with a great artist and gentleman whom I hold in high esteem. In fact, if I didn't value this noted imbiber so highly I probably would not have objected, violently in the end, to his repeated use of "Fuck you" while I was in conversation with an attractive young woman and his relentless insistence that I sign a petition on protecting the environment in Antarctica, a cause which I also supported.

I don't recall who struck the first blow, but I do remember being pulled off the artist when I had his ears in my hands and was attempting to bounce his skull off the floor. The amusing part was when another famous artist, a woman, began shouting, "Stop! Stop! We don't fight in the art world!" Really? Even at the time, that struck me as amusing. It seemed to me that fighting was a regular and vital part of the social life of the art world, especially during the halcyon days of Abstract Expressionism and bibulous debates at the Cedar Tavern. It was a way of standing by one's word.

Although casting aspersions is often considered a rationale or excuse for physical violence, I have found that the well-thought-out insult can often obviate more unpleasant and harmful forms of combat. Usually an argument leading to fisticuffs is public and has witnesses. If you can clearly best your opponent verbally in front of witnesses, ideally making the bystanders laugh, he will often slink away to think of a riposte. And the longer that process takes, the more futile any sort of retort becomes.

Aspersion must be extremely specific. If you're not specific it's not even an insult, and you are probably a bigot in the bargain. "Nigger!" "Faggot!" "Communist!" Oh, please! A good insult must be unique and descriptive, capturing the specific qualities in one's target that he most despises in himself, or, if you're really good, the flaws of which he was not entirely aware but may have suspected.

Most men employ a few stock epithets, giving no thought whatsoever to the pertinence or quality of their negative statements. "Asshole!" How original. "Scumbag!" Brilliant. Effective derision, the comment that really "gets 'em where they live," requires aptness and specificity.

The other important issue in combat is fear. Never show fear. Laugh in its face. Even if your heart is fluttering in your Egyptian-cotton shirt and the adrenaline is racing through your system, insisting that you flee, relax, smile, breathe. You will flee, of course, but at your own pace and on your own terms.

Flight is usually the best alternative to actual combat, but it should be disguised and never embarked upon in obvious haste. "Let's take this outside" is a traditional invitation to combat. Once outside, of course, away from onlookers, you have the option to attempt a quick getaway, to propose a negotiated compromise, or to offer a limited and qualified apology. But getaways can be triumphant: "If this taxi didn't happen to be coming, I'd thrash you senseless, if you weren't already senseless." A good departing line is key. It shows you aren't limited by archaic macho standards.

Of course, if one is faced with a formidable opponent, one can always suggest taking it outside, allowing your opponent to go first and then attempt to find an alternative egress. Years later you can always say, "Oh, you went out on the street? I was waiting in the alley! Another time, perhaps!"

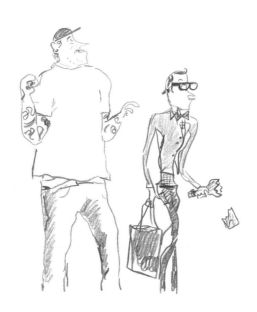

HOW TO HAVE A VICE

A vice is something you like to do that other people don't want you to do: drugs, drinking, smoking, gambling, sex outside the rules of the church and/or state. What they call a "bad habit." Sometimes vices are things we really enjoy. Sometimes they are things we enjoy even more because other people don't want us to do them. Sometimes they are things we enjoy, but feel guilty about.

But vice will go better all the way around if we understand it. And maybe give it a little love. It's only trying to help.

"Vice" comes from the Latin *vitium*, or fault, and it's the opposite of *virtus*, virtue. It's what makes you weak as opposed to what makes you strong, although sometimes we observe people who seem strengthened by their vices. We hear a lot about sobriety. We don't hear temperance discussed anymore. It's an old-fashioned virtue that seems to have been replaced by abstinence. "Temperance" means moderation, and we've lost sight of that old, conventional wisdom that says, "Everything in moderation." Now it's everything or nothing. That's no way to live. You've heard of tempered steel. They take that red-hot blade and plunge it into something cold. Well, maybe you can do something similar to your brain or your character. I say, take what you need. Temper yourself, by all means. But watch out for those who would mind your business for you.

Stamping out vice is one of the government's favorite purviews because it makes the enforcers feel righteous, and it makes lots of people rich on both sides of the illegal coin. Without narcotics there are no narcs. But the prohibition of activities enjoyed by significant minorities (or even the majority) can be misleading. Sometimes it's not about the vice but who enjoys it. Recent studies of the prohibition of alcohol in the United

States in the twenties have shown that the Eighteenth Amendment really had more to do with ethnic hatreds than alcohol.

White Anglo-Saxon Protestants, whose power was waning in the early twentieth century, associated the use of alcohol with immigrants, Catholics, Jews, and blacks, all groups with a higher birthrate. These WASPs were allied with feminist groups, including the Women's Christian Temperance Union and the Anti-Saloon League. There was also considerable anti-German sentiment involved as prohibitionists made much of German control of the American beer industry, and the Eighteenth Amendment was passed in the year following the end of the First World War. In fact, prohibition resulted not from a clear majority of teetotalers but from a coalition of haters.

Anti-marijuana laws also resulted from ethnic prejudices. Marijuana does not seem to have done Louis Armstrong much harm, or, for that matter, me either, but it was seen by excitable legislators and religion addicts as pernicious due to its popularity among blacks, jazz musicians, and liberals. Finally, prohibition is breaking down somewhat now that there is considerable evidence that this fragrant and attractive plant, once one of the most important crops on earth as the source of a fiber more useful and earth-friendly than cotton, is of considerable and irreplaceable medical value.

The chief result of prohibition, whether of alcohol or other drugs, has been the extraordinary enrichment of the traffickers in illegal substances, whose revenues have not only been inflated by artificial scarcity but are also entirely tax-free. There is nothing better for organized crime than prohibition. Today we are at war in Afghanistan, fighting a guerrilla army supported principally by traffic in opium and its derivatives. Opium is the largest export of Afghanistan, accounting for seventy-five to ninety percent of the world's supply. If the prohibitions against opium were lifted, the Taliban and other terrorist and criminal organizations would lose their principal source of funds. This is an old story. The heroin epidemics of the United States have long been related to American foreign policy. In the sixties and seventies heroin production was centered in Southeast Asia, among anticommunists supported by the CIA. For decades, narco-traffickers in Latin America and their North American associates have reaped billions in profits, dwarfing the fortunes built during the bootlegging twenties and thirties in the United States. And intelligence agencies dealing in drugs don't really need legislatures to fund their operations when they can do it themselves without oversight.

The enlightened approach, both on a personal and local level as well as on a global level, is to prohibit prohibition. We have all known persons with problems involving alcohol and drugs of one kind or another, but I have had no experience with anyone being helped by prohibitions. Lately, the idea that treatment works far better than punishment has caught on in some areas, but that realization is too late, as far more lives have been ruined by jail sentences for drugs than by drugs themselves.

Twelve-step programs have saved plenty of lives and alleviated a lot of suffering, but they are not the answer for everything. I think we have to deal with so-called vices culturally. Anonymous programs are religious, although they claim they are not. An integral part of the program is the admission of powerlessness and the acceptance of a higher power. Reason doesn't seem to count as one of those, although God, in any guise, does. I think reason is the highest power we have and by using it, you can have power over anything.

America's biggest drug problems are caused by the prohibition of drugs and by the pharmaceutical rocket scientists who always make things worse. Methadone, the most addictive of drugs, was invented as a cure for heroin. Heroin was invented as a cure for morphine addiction, and morphine was invented as a cure for opium addiction. Nobody had a coca-leaf problem until they invented cocaine. The bit of cocaine in the original Coca-Cola was not a big social problem. It was probably a good dosage. Picked you up. Coca-leaf chewers don't have problems. Cocaine is too strong, but scientists always want that "active ingredient," never appreciating the genius of nature. And then when the narcs made the chemicals used to refine cocaine hard to obtain, the dealers had a good idea: crack. Smoking it, nobody would notice that foul taste.

The derivatives of opium that are considered dangerous were all invented as cures for opium, which tends to make people sleepy. And marijuana…well, nobody got shot over it before it was illegal, and nobody had a problem with it until they discovered that THC is the "active ingredient" and growers began sex-starving their crop to maximize this in relation to the other phenolic compounds present in the natural plant. Now people are powerless over pot too. Oh, wow! If you are powerless over marijuana, you may have trouble with hot sauce.

While there are undoubtedly persons who are allergic to alcohol and who lose control under its influence, the positioning of alcoholism and drug addiction as diseases, and the subsequent inclusion of sexual compulsion, gambling compulsion, and chronic indebtedness has had unfortunate consequences. Charging too much on your MasterCard is now called a disease and sudden gambling sprees are listed as side effects of certain medications. All the more reason to keep the doctors away from issues of vice.

Gambling and drugs have been with us forever, and that won't change. Much of America's gambling difficulty is the result of credit problems encouraged by the crooks running our economic system. Gambling is part of our diseased culture. Today the stock market is modeled on Las Vegas. And poor Americans vote for tax breaks for the rich because they have that gambler's mentality. They plan to win the lottery.

Personally, I think gambling is stupid unless you are betting on yourself in a game of skill, in which case my advice is never give more than two strokes a side. Substances are a private matter. I'm not going to quibble with people's appetites, as long as they don't jeopardize others. Vice should be regulated by manners.

It is the height of rudeness to put another in jeopardy with one's state of mind, or with the possession of contraband. It is against the laws of hospitality to covertly introduce illicit commodities to another's premises. You should not be invited back. It is especially rude to shoot heroin in the powder room. What is more of an imposition than forcing your host to revive you as you turn blue? Only the disposal of your lifeless body.

HOW TO DRINK

"*Pithecanthropus erectus* was a teetotaler, but the angels, you may be sure, know what is proper at 5 PM."

—H. L. Mencken

"The only cure for a real hangover is death."

—Robert Benchley

Keith Richards named his personal band the X-pensive Winos after he caught them swigging Château Lafite as "light refreshment." This is an appellation I can relate to, because for the last decade or so I have more or less limited my consumption of alcohol to wine. I'm a wino with a vintage chart. It's not that I have taken a modified pledge or anything. I have at least one margarita annually, the occasional Dark and Stormy (ginger beer with rum), and a blue moon beer, but after many years of trial-and-error imbibing, I came to the conclusion that I was better off sticking with the wine.

In the nineties I drank a considerable amount of Belgian beer. I loved Duvel, which approaches wine in strength at 8.5 percent, and I liked a raspberry or peach Lambic ale now and then. Some Belgians I drank for the name, like Mort Subite (although it's great beer), Judas, Lucifer, Sublime, and Satan. If I have a beer now, I'll take a Stella Artois. But I essentially gave up beer because I did not want to weigh 230 pounds. No matter what anyone tells you, there is nothing more fattening than beer.

I also went wino because I came to believe it was compatible with evolution. Humans have been drinking wine since prehistory, whereas we've been drinking distilled spirits for less than a thousand years. From this I speculate that the human liver has had thousands of years more time to adapt to the wine habit. The alcohol level isn't as prodigious as booze. I am not sure that evolution has yet provided us with the enzymes and antibodies required to deal with spirits that are forty to fifty percent alcohol, but somehow I'm confident that my body can handle a liter of Barolo. I also know from experience that it's far easier to go too far with booze than wine, particularly if you tend to confuse thirst with Thirst. Tequila shots? That's OK, darling, I'll drive.

Another thing about spirits—I know that the sophisticated palette is supposed to like Scotch, Cognac, and eaux-de-vie. It's an acquired taste, they say, whereas I remember my grandma giving me a sip of her beer as a toddler and liking it instantly: Mmm, beer good! More! I also remember thinking wine wasn't so good. Later I realized that the wine I sipped was probably from a vineyard on Lake Erie.

Wine tastes good—even great. But if you have to put fruit juice in something, or if it's "an acquired taste," maybe you are fooling yourself. I did go through a brief period of drinking Scotch about twelve years ago, but that was because I realized that if I drank it I would never have more than one.

My grandfather, in whatever heavenly lounge he may be frequenting now, might be disappointed that I have grown gray without ever finishing a martini, but he'd give me credit for sticking to my guns. He gave me my first sips of Château d'Yquem and Château Haut-Brion, the oldest Bordeaux château, which he told me was founded by an O'Brien. A famous fib. But they can't deny that Lynch-Bages was made by an Irishman.

As a bartender and drinker, I did learn the intricacies of Scotch, bourbon, Cognac, rum, and vodka, as well as a bit about gin and tequila.

And I don't mean to suggest that drinkers of these liquors are wrong. Maybe they have more evolved livers than I do. I prefer to drink like an old Roman or Greek.

I have noted that many of the roués of the thirties, forties, and fifties seemed to have aged and died considerably younger than my generation. One might suspect that the death of Errol Flynn at fifty, Humphrey Bogart at fifty-seven, John Barrymore at sixty, and W. C. Fields at sixty-six had something to do with their prodigious consumption of spirits. Of course, we must remember that the spirits they consumed were illicit, and so there was no way of knowing the condition of the bathtub where their gin originated. Not to mention the heavy consumption of unfiltered coffin nails. No, there is no moral judgment in my wino lifestyle. It's a matter of taste, hangover minimization, and longevity.

When I first embarked on the wino lifestyle, I even attempted to drink the fruit of the vine as the Romans did, diluted with water. I only did this with white wine—it would spoil a good red—but most of us have enjoyed a spritzer and that is how the Romans drank—without the ice or bubbles, of course. (Although if they had Alpine snow they may have had spritz with that, up north around the Rubicon.)

In some classic literature, drinking full-strength wine is referred to as drinking "Scythian style." The Scythians, of course, were equestrian, trouser-wearing nomads considered relatively uncivilized, so this was not a chic practice. (Neither, we may assume, was their habit of throwing hemp flowers on the campfires until laughter broke out.) There is something to be said for spritzers when one is making a long evening of it, but after the summer, I resort to Scythian-style imbibing, which is really the only way to go with serious vintages, like the Falernian that Catullus praised (Aglianico), singing, "Begone, water, away with you, water, destruction of wine... "). In any case, I still try to drink a glass of water for every glass of wine. They mix inside.

Serious vintages are a good way of keeping oneself from overindulging, at least if money matters. I find that if I'm drinking a bottle of Château

L'Angélus or Ducru-Beaucaillou, I'm less likely to open that second bottle and then cork the leftover half. If I do cork the rest I know I'll feel guilty in the AM, so I'll probably drain the second bottle instead.

I have also observed that if I drink a nice full-bodied red, I will drink less. I love white wine, especially in the summer, but there's something about white that makes you keep drinking it. I used to think it was a blood-sugar thing, but maybe there's something in red that makes one mellow. White is more high-energy hilarity. At least, that's the way it seems with the ladies who lunch. Maybe it's a demon in me, but I genuinely believe that a good vintage is the finest form of health food.

The distillation of alcohol—a scientific breakthrough attributed to the Arabs and prized by alchemists and physicians—led to the creation of Cognac, whiskey, vodka, tequila, and all of the drinks we know as spirits, as well as a wide variety of liquors and liqueurs whose origins are in herbal medicine, such as Fernet-Branca. Today liquor is not often taken for medicinal purposes without irony, but it's nice to have a medicinal drink now and then, like vermouth or Chartreuse, an elixir for long life concocted of 130 herbs by the Carthusian monks.

Sometimes I wonder if the cultural enthusiasm for liquor as a daily source of alcohol, which peaked in the fifties and sixties before the wine revival and microbrew movement, is related to the great fallacy of the active ingredient. It's about cocaine not the coca leaf, heroin not opium, and grain alcohol not Vinho Verde. Scientists are always looking for that one thing in the ancient potion that does the trick, but there's the trick. The best remedies and potions are complex. Synthesis even ruined pot. I remember a kinder, gentler herb before scientifically inclined marijuana growers began to believe scientists' statements that THC was the "active ingredient" in cannabis and disregarded other ingredients such as CBD, which gave rise to the sinsemilla industry and turned the naturally benevolent herb into something resembling what its enemies claimed it was.

Nothing is as simple as we are led to believe. Go for complexity. It's good for you. Today we are finding more and more claims for wine's healthy properties, such as its antioxidant effect. Maybe it's time we start believing that old Bacchus knew a thing or two.

Drinking Tips

Decanting can't hurt. Oxygen brings many wines to a livelier life with a little time. And I really hate picking a big chunk of sediment out of my teeth.

Tasting the wine in a restaurant is not pretentious. It's important, since if they pour it, you pay for it. As much as eight percent of the wines sealed with actual cork are corked—that is, they are tainted by a fungus that gives the wine an unpleasant, musty odor and taste. A trained nose can pick it up before actually tasting the wine. Usually wine that comes in a screw-cap or synthetically corked bottle is going to be good, but it's still a good idea to taste it, as wines can also be ruined by exposure to heat or light. Don't feel sorry for the little establishment that pours you a bad bottle; they'll get their money back from the distributor. We don't send back a wine simply because we don't like it, although a server will probably take back something you don't like that he urged you to try. (And he'll drink it himself later.)

If you have only one thing in the refrigerator, make it Champagne. You'll be ready to celebrate or seduce at all times. And if you don't drink anything else you probably won't get a hangover. When popping Champagne, hold the bottle straight up lest you pop an eye out.

A gentleman keeps his eye on the ladies' glasses to make sure they are filled.

If you order white wine in a restaurant and it's not cold enough, dump the contents of a saltshaker into the ice bucket and mix well.

It is considered bad luck by some to pour one's own sake. It's romantic to take turns pouring.

If one is toasting or just saying "cheers," clink glasses gently with each member of the party while making eye contact with them, even if it is not returned. It's an old Italian custom designed to alert you if someone is trying to poison you. Clink and then drink, for God's sake. You can't clink and fail to imbibe immediately.

You can't really toast with water. Sorry.

If you know you're going to swig heavily, get a ride to the party and save yourself the trouble and notoriety of picking up your car the next day. You should not drink and drive. Or drink and send e-mails, or leave phone messages, or go on eBay.

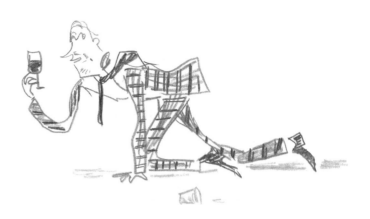

HOW TO SMOKE

"You die your way and I'll die mine."

—Frank Sinatra

My mother has lung cancer. She's eighty-seven. She's had the big C for several years now, but she's holding her own. She's also had emphysema for many years. She hasn't had a cigarette in ten years, but she does have a carton of Parliaments stashed in her kitchen drawer in case there's a nuclear war.

My mom started smoking at sixteen because she thought it looked glamorous. She started out with Lucky Strikes, which came in a handsome little package. When I was little, she smoked Chesterfields. When filters became the fashion, she switched to Parliaments—I'm guessing for the recessed filter. They advertised "maximum health protection."

When I was a boy and I got an earache, my grandpa used to blow smoke in my ear. His folk medicine made me feel better. He smoked Camels that he kept in a leather box. I liked the way it smelled and the way he smelled—bay-rum cologne and tobacco. Later he switched from Camels to Kents, probably for the "Micronite filter" that Kents enthusiastically advertised. It later turned out that the Micronite filter contained crocidolite, a particularly dangerous form of asbestos.

My brother still smokes Camels. His fingers are brown at the tips. He says they calm him down. My stepfather smoked Old Golds. He probably liked the long legs of the girls in the dancing cigarette packs. Their slogan was: "No song and dance about medical claims. Old Gold's specialty is to give you a treat instead of a treatment." He quit when he retired, and he passed away last spring at eighty-nine. I think it was the way they treated him in the hospital that killed him, not the cigs. I'm sure he smoked because it made the time pass at work, just as they did when he was in combat on a battleship in the Pacific and the smoking lamp was lit. Most guys smoked when the smoking lamp was lit.

I grew up in a world that smoked. There was no place I would rather be than in a nightclub, even as a kid, if I could con my folks into taking me along. I loved to watch a jazz band, drink a Roy Rogers fake cocktail, and bask in the smoky atmosphere. Of course it was smoky at home too. If there were such a thing as secondhand smoke, I would have died long ago. My mother was smoking with me at her breast.

I smoked on and off for years, although I haven't had a cigarette or cigar going on seven years. In Venice recently, I had a dessert with tobacco in it but I didn't get off on it. I still get a yen for a cigarette sometimes, usually if I'm at the beach, but I'm done with it. When I'm working out or have a winter cough, I wish I'd never, ever smoked.

A few years ago I had a noncancerous growth removed from my gum, right where I used to clench a Marlboro red when I was typing. A few months ago, a wealthy cigar aficionado handed me a very valuable pre-Castro Cuban after dinner. I put it in my pocket, and he said, "Aren't you going to smoke it?" I said, "Yeah, but I'm saving it for my deathbed."

For years, I had an old lady physician who smoked one cigarette a day, after dinner. "Big deal," she said. I agree. I was never really hooked except once when I took up Camel straights for an extended period. I was in the Hamptons and my car was in the shop. It was raining and I ran out of Camels. I found a pack of Marlboro lights and smoked one, but nothing happened. I smoked another—nothing. I needed a Camel. Their old slogan was "I'd walk a mile for a Camel," and I wound up literally walking a mile for a Camel. But then I didn't really have any trouble quitting. It's willpower. But that concept doesn't fit in with the culture of powerlessness that has taken over in America. It's a disease!

Or is it just giving up, denying responsibility? The Marlboro Man made me do it. If it never occurred to you that spending a large part of your life sucking on hot fumes from burning leaves and inhaling them deeply into your lungs might not be good for you, then you are a fool and nobody made you that but yourself. On the other hand, if, like my old doctor, you like a single taste of the ancient American Indian herb after dinner, well, cheers!

Smoking tobacco was not always considered a vice. Native to the Americas, tobacco was used religiously by American Indians. Among eastern North American tribes, it was extensively traded and smoked ceremonially on significant occasions. The value placed on tobacco by the natives piqued the interest of Europeans, who brought it back to the Continent as early as the late fifteenth century. It caught on immediately as a medicine and as a recreational drug. As late as the 1940s, tobacco was promoted for its beneficial properties. One campaign advised people to smoke Camels for their health. Another had the family dentist recommending Viceroys.

I don't smoke. I'm not for it, but I'm not against it. I'm for freedom, and I don't like the way the nonsmoking majority has demonized the smoking minority. We've all seen people react to someone lighting a cigarette as though the smoker were lighting a match next to a running gas pump. It's a form of hysteria, and that hysteria has reached mass proportions. Secondhand smoke probably has no effect whatsoever except on certain people who have allergies, as they might to cats or pollen. What about secondhand cats? Secondhand ragweed?

I don't really believe there is such a thing as secondhand smoke, any more than there are secondhand farts or secondhand car exhaust. Well, I guess there is secondhand car exhaust from secondhand cars. But I doubt that secondhand smoke has ever killed anyone. Scientists have been paid handsomely to fabricate arcane statistics to suggest that someone smoking a Winston one hundred yards downwind will probably induce emphysema in you by morning, but these are the same sort of researchers who are suggesting that radioactive hamburger is healthier than plain. If secondhand smoke were dangerous, my mother would have killed me by the time

I was ten. Let's face it, the worst thing secondhand smoke can do is increase your dry-cleaning bill and require more frequent shampooing.

I am not suggesting that smoking is harmless. Smoking isn't a yogic breathing exercise. Smoke too much and you die. I am not suggesting that the tobacco industry is blameless or that it has not been guilty of criminal acts. But lots of businesses have been guilty of criminal acts. What happened to tobacco is a lot like what happened to food and alcoholic beverages. Industrialization and commerce have a tendency to ruin things once held sacred. We have tobacco criminals, and we have corn criminals, meat criminals, milk criminals, and fruit and vegetable criminals. How many do you think will ever be brought to justice unless karma plays hardball?

The U.S. government has approved 599 additives for use in the manufacture of cigarettes—additives that keep them fresh longer, keep them burning, boost the nicotine kick, and dilate the airway, and additives to alter the taste of what is sometimes inferior tobacco. While all these additives were tested for safety when in food, none of them were tested for burning. So if there's crime afoot, hasn't the government been complicit?

One interesting response to the fear of tobacco was the creation of Natural American Spirit cigarettes, which use whole-leaf tobacco containing no additives. Two of the ten varieties offered by the company are made from organic tobacco. But in line with a Federal Trade Commission ruling, American Spirits carry a warning that their product is as hazardous as other cigarettes are. Hmm. What about the ones with the artificial "flavor" sprayed on?

Shouldn't there be bars and restaurants where consenting adults can smoke cigarettes? Where they can be free from hysterics who fear death from their neighbor's next exhale? Why do we need so much protection from ourselves? I guess it's to give the authorities work.

All the evidence I have left is in Genesis: "Of every tree of the garden thou mayest freely eat: but of the tree of the knowledge of good and evil, thou shalt not eat of it; for in the day that thou eatest thereof thou shalt surely die." I'm not sure what that means, but if it means that God granted man dominion over plants, maybe we should reconsider banning tobacco. Men spent millions of years learning the magical secrets of plants. Then science spent a few decades learning how to pervert them, giving us crack, smack, and True low-tar cigarettes. If it is science against the shaman, sometimes you just have to leave the glittering citadel of science and head back to the jungle for a breath of fresh smoke.

I will probably never smoke another cigarette or cigar, but if a tribal elder offered me a hit on the pipe, well, what visions might come? The American Indians used tobacco in an entirely different manner from the white man, as a shamanic sacrament. I'm down with that. Vision is in short supply now. And who can say how magic works? Who's going to tell Jean-Paul Belmondo, "Put down that Gitane"?

"Vous mourrez votre façon. Je mourrai le mien."

Next thing you know, they'll be outlawing oral sex. Oh, wait, I guess that's already illegal in some states. Must be people are worried about secondhand sex.

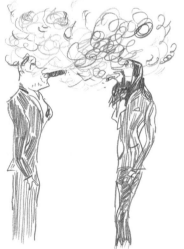

Smoking in Your Home

If you serve as host to smokers, whatever your own habits, it is a kindness to provide them with a civilized and not uncomfortable place to practice their legal and long-accepted habit. Not to mention an ashtray. If there's anything that makes me cringe, it's a friend leaning out the window, blowing smoke and steam into the frostbitten atmosphere. Anyone who makes their friends go outside to smoke a cigarette should not be permitted to watch Humphrey Bogart or Bette Davis movies.

I know there are many who believe smoking is a filthy, toxic habit, but one of the cleanest homes I know belongs to a friend who smokes at least a pack a day. He is a prodigious cleaner, however, and he knows all the tricks, including Carta d'Armenia papers from Farmaceutica di Santa Maria Novella in Firenze, imbued with the scent of frankincense and myrrh and benzoin to remove unpleasant odors from the air. Many of the agitators who live in horror of cigarettes reside alongside overflowing cat boxes, matted Labrador retrievers, and unscrubbed trash cans. Let he who is without odor cast the first aspersion.

Lighting Up as a Visitor

If you still smoke, you have probably been trained by now to skulk outside to light up. There are, however, civilized folk among us who are reasonable and kind. There is no reason to assume you will not be permitted to smoke and I, for one, would prefer that you ask if you may smoke before heading out the window and occupying the fire escape.

The Japanese make a nice little portable ashtray, or *keitai haizara*. Disposing of your own butts will give the world one less reason to deny you.

Chewing

If you chew tobacco, do it at home, alone, or with others who practice your vile vice. Or in a field somewhere. Like Elvis, the spittoon has left the building.

HOW TO HAVE A HOME

"If you didn't have so much stuff, you wouldn't need a house. You could just walk around all the time."

—George Carlin

Just because a man's home is his castle doesn't mean it has to be cold, dark, and sparsely furnished. Maybe a castle is too limiting. How about a man's home is his palace? Yeah, that's more like it.

My palace isn't just a place for me to hang my crown; it's also a place where my consort and my heirs can hang their crowns, and we can hold court, full court, or half-court. It's a place for feasting with my loyal retainers and my peers. It's a place I can furnish befitting my station and display my treasures for the world to see. My palace lets the world know who I am and where I'm at. It's my territory. It's the seat of my power (not to mention my butt), a refuge against adversity (and assholes), a shelter from the storm (and the IRS), and a place to sleep, perchance to dream (or get a back rub). And as George Carlin said, "the meaning of life is finding a place for your stuff."

In this age of casual, homes are more the measure of a man than the clothes on his back. A man has his place, or he's the fugitive kind. Some men understand how a man is nurtured and fortified by his home, but many don't get it. They see their home simply as the crash pad. Or they see it as an ostentatious display of their wealth and celebrity taste, with all the comforts of the MTV Crib. Pity the fool who lives by wide-screen, lounge chair, and mattress alone. Fortune favors the man who knows how to live large in his large living room. By their McMansions ye shall know them.

Legions of Wall Street bonus babies have taken up with fancy decorators, hoping that taste professionals will help them flaunt an aura of personality that they are ill equipped to manifest unaided. But bold, fortunate, and resourceful is the man who does it himself, the man who is his own prop stylist, the man who has dug deep to find his own interior interior decorator.

The first step toward making a home is finding a suitable place. It may be large or small, depending on your needs and resources, but it should be appropriate and it should be in the right place. Location, location, location! The right place suits your style. It inspires you. And it may even provide some elements of community, a hard thing to find in cities. This is where instinct kicks in. You walk around, you drive around, and you come to a place that has the right look and the right feel. You almost feel at home. (Except you haven't got your stuff with you.) It's like dowsing or finding water with a twig. You move and you move and then there you are. This must be the place. You are home. Home is you. Not them. You.

Some men go into stores with their girlfriends (or boyfriends, or mothers) with the intention of buying a new bed or chair and suddenly they develop narcolepsy. They mumble, "They all look the same...I don't know...you decide." This is your first and fatal error. You do have an opinion; it's in there, you just have to find it. To find your inner interior decorator, first you must find your inner control freak.

Look at each chair in the store and imagine someone is forcing it on you. Eventually one chair will say something to you: "I'm OK," maybe, or "I'm not hers; I'm yours." And then you have found your inner chair. And now you can begin to find a pattern of affinities. You begin to see: "These are things I can work with." Once you have begun to assert control over your surroundings you will begin to discover your taste, even if you thought you didn't have any. Don't worry if it seems bad at first—at least you've located it. You can trade up later.

Some men are reticent about asserting their taste because first they must realize that they need and deserve a home. You don't have to be a child, a roommate, or a guest all your life. A man doesn't have to have a live-in companion, wife, or children to deserve a home. Everyone deserves a home. If you're not sure, maybe reciting some New Age affirmations will help.

Repeat after me: "I am somebody. This is not my parents' house. This is *my* house."

I give my wife full credit for encouraging me to find my interior interior decorator. I was getting divorced and living in a new apartment in a fine old doorman building. I had a TV, a bed, and a desk made from a door and two sawhorses. In the apartment, I was drinking Belgian beer and watching TV. Although I had a good TV, I didn't even have a sofa to watch it from. Theoretically this might have made it easier to get girls into bed, but it was pathetic. My future wife knew that a major antiques show was coming up. "Let's go," she said.

We went. She didn't make any forward moves. She didn't say much. But eventually I found a coffee table that I liked, a modern, blond, round table. It spoke to me. I think it said "Good for holding beer and newspaper," but it also pleased me design-wise. It was $150. I thought that was too much. Considering my income level, this was absurd. I was psychologically blocked. So she said something profound.

"Would you spend that much for wine at dinner?"

"Sure," I said, knowing I had no chance of lying on that count.

"OK," she said, "You buy the table and I'll buy dinner."

Before I knew what hit me, I was antiquing every weekend.

I was buying things that suited the taste in furniture I didn't know I had. But you don't have to do it all yourself. Don't be the guy driving in strange territory who refuses to stop and ask for directions. It's OK to solicit advice, professional or otherwise. Find places where you feel comfortable and happy, and find out who made them that way. Read *The World of Interiors* and *Casa Vogue,* and discover just how far personality can assert itself in making a home.

Even for the most talented and committed do-it-yourself decorators, there are connoisseurs out there and shamans and scholars of the obscure who can enhance your own proclivities and educate your palette. Sometimes when you're stumped you need a consultant, a second opinion. I have allowed Mr. Ricky Clifton, for example, an artist, decorator, and intrepid shopper, to have several vodkas, smoke pot, and then move my furniture around. It's like attending a séance. Of course, a Ricky Clifton doesn't come around every lifetime, but if you find a friend who knows everything about the Meiji Restoration or the Aesthetic movement, or the difference between David Smith and Tony Smith and Harry Smith and Jack Smith, you should hold on to him.

Decor must be realistic. Nothing looks sillier than some big, fat CEO putting a delicate Chippendale bird's-eye maple chair at risk. A fat man needs big, steel chairs. Decoration is not abstract but specific. It should be about who inhabits the space. I will never forget visiting a famous writer about art. At first glance it appeared to be one of those supremely tasteful Upper East Side apartments, but looking more closely at the art and the "objets," I began to realize that many of them were on the theme of, well, let's say man's cruelty to man. I had the distinct impression that somewhere in this large apartment within shouting distance of the Frick Collection was a closet with a black leather motorcycle jacket in it. Antiques can be boring without a context, and a big personality provides big-time context. The refinement of a Louis XV chair stands out so much more when it's beside an iron maiden or a cuirass.

In other words, one's home should manifest one's tastes, interests, obsessions, and even peccadilloes. In my house you'll find a lot of art; Swedish modern furniture; R&B and reggae on vinyl; baseballs autographed by knuckleball pitchers; modern first editions; African masks and witch-doctor whistles; Raymor pottery; oriental rugs; photos of jazz musicians; a giant marble hand; a gold record; a leather rhinoceros footstool; and a framed restaurant napkin with a quote from Karl Marx written on it by Carl Andre in 1973. That's who I am, baby. Oh, and several thousand books.

There's something about our time that makes you wish that you lived in another one. And that's the great thing about antiques. Through them you *can* live in other times. We all have periods and places we admire for one reason or another, some cultural resonance that moves us. I agree with the great Italian designer Piero Fornasetti: "I do not believe in eras or times. I do not. I refuse to establish the value of things based on time."

My wife is still trying to eradicate my fondness for the Arts and Crafts movement. I have always liked the philosophy behind it and the aesthetics that combined a modest modernism and utopianism with fine do-it-yourself craftsmanship, and I still love the ginger-haired girls in those Pre-Raphaelite paintings, but I do understand my wife's problem with it. I bought my first Gustav Stickley piece decades ago, but now Stickley is so popular that fashion models own it. I've managed to hang on to a bookshelf and some vases, but I'm afraid to leave town for more than a week.

I also see Arts and Crafts as a hedge against our home being too midcentury modern. Why live in one style or period when you can live in several? Styles are powerful, so when one you love becomes dominant, you feel like giving up and moving on, lest you become part of the problem and not the solution. You don't want to be an adherent. If you're all of a period, it's like getting dressed head to toe by one designer. You become the collected not the collector.

I am pro-eclectic because there's something almost fascist about having a strict period thing going on. It's a problem I have with the current midcentury modern craze. If that's all there is, the atmosphere is too cool for school. The best room in *Mad Men* is the office of old Bert Cooper, a mix of modernist furniture with abstract art and Japanese antiques. It has depth. It's worldly.

In an eclectic context, each piece makes the others look more interesting because of the unexpected contrast. You need balance in your spaces. For me, the antidote to the totalitarianism of modernism is to stick something baroque or gothic into the mix, something that Morticia and Gomez Addams would have loved, a piece with a dragon's or gargoyle's head and claw feet, Victorian *faux bois* tables, or fanciful Chinese pieces made from burled roots.

Ultimately, successful decor is about genuine personal taste. It's fine for bachelors to have antique bowling pins, golf clubs, top hats, or ancient gin bottles, barber poles, and other things that might horrify a wife (or even me). A good Louisville Slugger collection is nothing to sneeze at. But it should be in its place, not too prominent. That makes you look nuts. A living room decorated with officially licensed sporting goods and jerseys is OK if you're thirteen but creepy if you're an adult. Remember, Adam Sandler is just playing those characters.

Also, as the old saying goes, books do furnish a room. And I'm not talking about fancy calf bindings with gilt titles; I'm talking about book jackets from the fifties and sixties. There's nothing like a real personal library, a rare thing in the Internet age. Our city place didn't have room for a separate library, so we combined it with the dining room. Now if dinner conversation lags, you can pick up a novel.

If you're going start furnishing your home, take a step back. You need to get a handle on the big picture. You have to visualize how things line up. Sometimes it's useful to draw your space and make small-scale cutouts of your furniture. It can save some heavy lifting.

Remember, people aren't going to just sit there; they are going to walk through rooms, sometimes with people sitting in them.

Visualize. Imagine the room with a great party in it. Imagine it with a naked girl in it. Is the room festive? Seductive? Mysterious? Loungeable?

Men must avoid bachelor mistakes, like centering a room around the television (unless it is clearly "the TV room") or centering your life on a Barcalounger. If your place looks like it was designed to watch football in, that's probably all that will ever happen there.

A mattress on the floor is not a bed. The sides of box springs should never be exposed to the view of women. You don't need a fancy bed frame, but get it up off the floor at least, and drape it. And don't ignore linens; go for a high thread count. That's not a myth; it's more quantifiable than IQ, and you spend a third of your life between the sheets.

The best way to avoid typical male lapses is to use your imagination: try seeing the place from a woman's point of view. If that's not working, invite some women over. Or visualize. Think, What would Kate Moss hate about this room? Where would Charlize Theron sit?

The plethora of furnishings enjoyed by my family (and if you look up "plethora," you'll realize that it means overabundance) has been accumulated in various ways. Some things were found at antiques stores, others at antiques fairs. Some things were discovered at yard sales. Some were purchased on eBay and at auction, both online and in the flesh.

I still love going into antiques stores, and when I say antiques, I don't necessarily mean things that are at least fifty years old, the technical definition. I'm talking about pre-owned stuff above the salvage level. I rarely buy something on the first visit to a shop unless I realize it's a steal that may be gone by the time I get back, even if it'll be the next day. My wife will never let me forget the pair of aluminum drum side tables that turned out to be worth ten times the asking price.

On the other hand, I believe that bargaining, as much as it goes against my instincts and natural-born-sucker sense of grandeur, is absolutely necessary. Getting something knocked off the asking price is expected and helps mitigate guilt later. I expect that anything I spot in an antique store can be had for at least twenty percent less than the tag says.

It's harder and harder to find bargains because more and more antique stores are aware of the market. Even mom-and-pop shops in out-of-the-way places are aware of what's selling for what in the big city, so don't expect a back-roads dealer to be a rube. He's on the Internet. Maybe you're shy of buying on the Web (and there is no substitute for seeing and touching the goods in person), but Internet auctions and online auction-house records can help you determine if a price is fair. I still go to book fairs, but these days it's always with a portable browser for checking prices on the Internet book marts. It's a little harder with furniture, but the information is there if you are a capable digger.

Antiques fairs are time saving because a big fair is the equivalent of maybe a hundred antiques shops, and you can get a sense of where the market is going. You might even get a bargain, particularly on the last day of the show, because dealers don't want to load it in the truck and schlep it back to the shop.

Wherever you choose to begin the refurbishment of your domicile, don't be blinded by atmosphere or caught up in the frenzy of money changing hands. Keep your head. Set some rules for yourself. Or borrow mine.

• Throw stuff out. Men have a bad habit of holding on to things, like ugly towels, stained sheets, and Grandma's toaster oven. Laziness and sentiment are the enemies of an inspired domicile.

• Don't hide the TV. Electronic stuff is part of our world. Let it be. I don't mind looking at your amp and turntable as long as good sounds are on. Just keep the wires neat.

• A good education can be had from *Antiques Roadshow.*

• Take Bruno's advice and don't get too "matchy matchy." Your mother needed a dining room set, but you can have six different chairs at your dinner table as long as they are really good chairs.

• A cart or table covered in liquor bottles? A piano covered in small silver-framed photographs? Give me a break. You might as well leave the Social Register next to the toilet.

• Fresh flowers liven up the place. Don't mix them if you don't know what you're doing. The guy at the deli definitely doesn't know what he's doing.

• It's cool to mix expensive stuff with cheap stuff, as long as the cheap is good quality. There's nothing wrong with mixing antiques you bought at auction with serviceable stuff from West Elm, Crate & Barrel, or Design Within Reach. But it's better to have one beautiful, expensive thing than ten cheap things. You've got your whole life ahead of you.

• Feng shui rules are OK as long as they make sense—like ensuring that the bed is accessible from two sides if you want to get a girlfriend. Some of the rules are insane, like having a beaded curtain instead of a bedroom door. As a man with children, let me tell you, you want a door that locks. We're not in China anymore, Dorothy.

• Posters of sports stars or kittens doing funny things should be avoided whenever possible.

• The light in the bathroom should be as good as in a dermatologist's office. Avoid hairy ears, bad shaves, and melanoma.

• Irony is permissable, but kitsch is death. I don't just mean collecting cheesecake postcards or lawn jockeys or Santa figurines. I mean being too fifties, or too forties. Or collecting bad religious art, like 3-D crucifixes. Humor has its place, but you don't want to live in a fun house.

• Don't be afraid to fill your house with beautiful and inspiring things. I never really lost money because I never bought stocks. I don't understand financial instruments. I do understand chairs.

• If you have a living room, live in it. This isn't the sixties and you're not your parents. Don't save things for company; you are the company.

• If you don't love it, don't buy it.

• If you like something in an antique store and are shocked by the price, don't be afraid to ask about it. Write down the names and dates and do some research—the Internet makes this easy. You may discover it is a bargain after all, or find it somewhere else cheaper. If nothing else, you'll know more about the market.

• Sofas are crucial in the male domain. They are often the centerpiece to one's living room and are generally crucial to spectator sports, reading, seduction, foreplay, and napping. What insomniac can resist a good sofa and the *New York Times* crossword? I always have a sofa in a bedroom. (We have a small recamier in a bathroom that's good for putting on your socks.) Sofas are also handy for very brief extended family accommodations.

The worst decor bullying I ever took was when I let my wife give away a supremely comfortable white denim–slipcovered down-filled sofa. She gave it away to a now-famous actress who gave it away soon afterward when she left for Hollywood. It was the perfect napping spot, and I sometimes wonder who's snoozing on it now. Every man should have a den of his own. A place for his stuff. Men in couples should, in fact, exercise special care when it comes to selecting a sofa; you may wind up sleeping on it.

HOW TO BE A HOST

One of life's great pleasures is entertaining friends and acquaintances on your own turf. It's a way of demonstrating your philosophy of life— how things ought to be—and learning something in the process.

The role of the host is ancient and sacred. In earlier times the home was not just a pad or a crib but a refuge against a hostile and unaccommodating world.

In ancient Greece, hospitality was a vital and sacred aspect of culture. If a stranger came by and you didn't wash him up, wine him, and dine him before asking his name and where he was coming from and where he was going, Zeus would not be pleased with you. Furthermore, the visitor was to feel safe inside your door in case the Man came knocking. The same standard of hosting was upheld in ancient Rome. If a potential host didn't kill you right off, he was likely to prove most accommodating. Similar notions of hospitality have been key elements of culture in the Middle East, in India, and in Celtic societies, where they'd side with a guest against a hostile clan, a posse, or the police.

The key of hospitality is to make your guests feel at home in that ancient sense: comfortable, safe, at ease. And in today's world of iffy standards, providing true hospitality can transform your guest's entire concept of living by providing an extraordinary example. A great host transcends mere duty, honoring his guests and elevating an ordinary occasion to new heights of celebration and enjoyment. And, fortunately, you no longer have to wash your guests' feet or shield them from the heat.

Dinner

One of the most enjoyable aspects of home life is the meal cooked in your kitchen, served at your table, and appreciated by your friends.

The most important part of a dinner party is the party, not the dinner. Dinner is important, but a year later you're going to remember everyone talking about the biggest lie they ever told, not how the roast turned out. Dinner is the highest form of socializing. It's where great conversation happens and where intimacy develops naturally and delightfully. There's something sacramental about breaking bread with friends, old or new. And if you're the host, you don't have to drive home.

The best dinner parties mix people who know each other and people who don't. Drawing up a good guest list is part instinct and part logic. The instinct part is about speculative interpersonal chemistry—you suspect A might like B, while C and D might find each other hotly simpatico. The logic is in assembling a balanced group. It's almost like putting together a team for a pickup game. You want somebody who can shoot, somebody who can pass, and somebody who can clear the boards. At a dinner party you want somebody who can be provocative, somebody who can enchant, and someone who can get laughs. Of course, you don't want a fist-fight or impromptu adultery, but you do like things to be lively. Thus the host is not simply a passive provider, the maître d', chef, and sommelier; a good host is also the leader of the conversation, the talk-show meister who prevents dead air, the helmsman who steers away from rocky subjects, the parliamentarian who keeps conversation civil and above board, the Heimlich giver, the Solomonic arbiter, and the nimble subject changer.

If a desired guest is half of a couple, you have to invite the other half too—unless you can figure out when he will be out of town. If you invite a single, let him bring a date. Sometimes that surprise guest adds a magical x factor that makes things work. Do arrange a seating plan: boy, girl, boy, girl.

The host and hostess, or host and host, should sit at the table's head and foot and put the guests of honor at their right. Put people who don't know each other together. Do not seat couples together. Couples are conversation killers, and the shy one will want to take the easy way out. If they try to sit together, stop them. In fact, separate them as far as possible. If a nervy wife tries to corral her husband, seat him next to the cutest girl. Never let a guest subvert your plan, which is based on who should meet whom, and which pair makes the most promising comedy team. The liveliest dinners are probably those where people who misunderstand or fear each other wind up lifelong pals, where treaties are brokered, and where love affairs bloom. "You're getting a divorce?" "Yeah, remember that dinner you gave last August?" That's good hosting. Remember, you're not just planning a dinner party; you're changing the world.

Overnight Guests

A big closet does not make a guest room. If you have a guest room, it should have breathing room, a comfortable bed, and all the amenities that your own bedroom contains—an alarm clock, extra pillows and blankets, drinking water, flowers, a good book or two, etc.

The guest bathroom should also have all the necessities—including a blow-dryer, new toothbrushes, toothpaste, disposable razors, cotton balls and swabs, shampoo and conditioner, Band-Aids, disinfectants, and antibiotic cream. It is nice to provide bathrobes and all the other amenities one would expect in a first-class hotel, excepting, of course, chocolates on the pillow. Books, as they say, do furnish a room and I like to provide a substantial selection for guests. Sometimes I edit what's in the room. I might take out the three-volume set of Russ Meyer's memoirs and replace it with a selection of Dave Barry and Dan Jenkins.

A guest room need not have a television, although it can be useful if your guests happen to show up with their children, in which case a stash of kiddie videos, from *Teletubbies* to *SpongeBob*, will help keep them occupied. If you have a swimming pool, keep a range of swimsuits available for men, women, and children.

The host need not provide condoms, lubricants, a dildo, or tranquilizers, but it's good to have an over-the-counter pain reliever and antacid on hand, in case your guests enjoy dinner excessively. My pain reliever of choice is ibuprofen, as acetaminophen is rough on the liver and aspirin can lead to million-dollar lawsuits when guests' children somehow develop Reye's syndrome. And it's an anti-inflammatory, which I interpret as "food for a hangover."

Make sure that your guests can have coffee if they are early risers. There's no obligation for you to get up at dawn just because they do. Before bed, I announce that I tend to luxuriate on the weekends, and I show where the tea, coffee, and decaf are and how to work the excellent Bunn coffeemaker, and where the thermos is, should there be one decaf and one high-test drinker. I will eventually make them breakfast, sometime before lunch, but in the meantime I show where the fruit, juices, baked goods, and other fixings can be found.

If you live in the country and dinner guests manage to become too intoxicated to drive home safely, and there is no one else available and sober enough to see to it, show them to the guest room. Their embarrassment in the morning will be worth it. If you allow them to take their chances, remember that some benighted jurisdictions hold hosts criminally liable for the poor driving of impaired guests.

Pets should be agreed upon beforehand, not a surprise, and if you allow them they must abide by your house rules. Just because they are permitted to mount the furniture at home doesn't give them the right to plop on the Wegner sofa *chez vous*. I am amazed by the number of friends who have arrived for a weekend with an unexpected and usually incontinent animal. On one occasion, I came close to covert canicide. On another—well, let's just say that cur lives on in memory. Be careful to close the door to the basement where the rat poison is deployed.

Even worse than a poorly behaved dog—and I'm not counting cats, to which my door is eternally barred due to allergy—is a badly behaved child, because no matter how awful it is, it is still a human and one's options are not quite so open. Toys are required for children, and it's good to keep some around, even if you have no offspring of your own. Board games are good as are large plastic vehicles with no small parts. Problem children will always find a way to swallow or inhale small objects, so never allow them to play with toys they may deliberately mistake for food or air. Again, television can be a godsend, as most children are addicted to it and will watch utter dreck for hours. And while I have certain regrets over purchasing a video-game system for my son, I have taken some mischievous delight in passing on this incurable addiction to the obstreperous children of guests.

Having guests can be its own reward. Your wife is far more likely to be on her best behavior with other people around. Your children, who are bored with you, will be kept busy. And people who only know you from your behavior at the office will be pleased to learn that you indeed have human qualities. But guests are not all fun, all the time. They have moods, allergies, illnesses, and weaknesses that you may be unaware of. Or connections you are aware of. I happen to be blessed with wonderful in-laws, but I am always aware that their presence increases the distaff scrutiny of my behavior.

And then, we will always have *The Man Who Came to Dinner*—or for those who have not seen the seminal 1942 comedy of hospitality run amok, starring immortals Bette Davis and Monty Woolley, that guest who it seems will never leave and whose stay tests the limits of one's endurance. The better the experience you provide for your guests, the more likely it is that some of them will forget that they are not a part of your family and attempt to, if not move in, considerably extend their visit. The odds of this happening increase, as I well know, if you live in a picturesque area, especially near a beach or ski slope.

As Benjamin Franklin wrote in *Poor Richard's Almanack* (1736): "Guests, like fish, begin to smell after three days." Modern refrigeration has not changed the truth of this maxim. It is always those guests with whom time flies, who are a delight to host, actually leave the place cleaner than it was when they arrived, and know precisely when to go, who in fact leave a bit on the early side, so that you actually feel a little lonely for ten or fifteen minutes after they have departed. The rotten guests are the ones who are wide awake and yapping, helping themselves to another bottle of your '95 St. Julien when you are yawning after having cooked and served the dinner and done the dishes. It is usually at this midnight hour that you learn about their discovery that something extraordinary is going on in your community just the day after they are scheduled to leave. Or that they have taken such a shine to the area that they want to stay to visit a local real estate agent. They are daring you to eighty-six them, knowing that you are probably far too kind.

It is always prudent to agree on the exact terms of a visit before a guest's arrival. This will save discomfort and embarrassment later. Alterations can be made, but if there is a departure date and time set you can always announce the imminent arrival of Aunt Fredegonde and her six special-needs refugee children.

It never hurts to have a train or bus schedule in the guest room, where it can be easily found, as well as a list of key telephone numbers—say, the local taxi and limousine services, and better inns and bed-and-breakfasts.

HOW TO BE A GUEST

It's an affirmation of the esteem in which you are held to have the pleasure of your company requested, whether it's for lunch, cocktails, dinner, dancing, or a weekend in the country. So don't fuck it up. Being a guest is not a free ride. You may not have to sing for your supper and you may believe that your good looks and charm are enough to justify your membership in the party, but there are still duties incumbent upon the guest, and if these are seen to with alacrity, you will find yourself in demand as a guest of honor. Or at least as the extra guy.

Dinner

When you are invited to dinner, remember to RSVP so that there are no mistakes. Failing to do so makes you a de facto crasher. Don't assume you are invited to bring a date, unless the invitation is clearly for you and your significant other, or you and a guest. If there's any doubt, clear it up early.

As a dinner guest, it is good form to bring a gift along for the host or hostess. Wine is almost always welcome, except in the homes of some sober alcoholics. (No doubt you will know if your friends are the sort who can't keep it in the house, in which case they probably shouldn't be entertaining anyway, except members of their own fraternity.) Bring something good; don't cheap out. It is not expected that the wine you bring will be served at dinner, as you probably don't know what's on the menu and your bottle might not be the best accompaniment to the chow. I have felt disappointment at seeing my Domaine des Tempiers go unopened, but that's show business. In my experience, however, cold Champagne is quite likely to be popped.

I have heard of people who are rude enough to repossess wine they had brought to a dinner. A person exhibiting such egregiously mingy behavior was once called an Indian giver, a peculiar term considering that the Indians were generally the ones whose things were taken away. As "The Word Detective" Evan Morris has noted: "The victors in history usually get to make up the idioms." Perhaps a better modern term for someone who gives something and later takes it back, after nearly everyone has gone home, would be "congressman."

A dinner guest can also bring a little gift of any sort. Some guests bring flowers. I have done it myself, even though I know this is frowned upon by some decor dictators. I figure that if the flowers are nice and the host doesn't like them for the table, they can go in the second guest bathroom.

Like houseguests, dinner guests shouldn't overstay their welcome. I find that at a congenial gathering of cool people, everyone leaves at about the same time. If everyone else is hitting the road, you should probably hit it too, unless the host begs you to stay. And I mean begs. Better they should miss you than have them yawning and clock-watching.

Eat what you are fed and don't complain. If you keep kosher or halal, your hosts probably know and will take this into consideration. If you are on a macrobiotic diet, I have it on good authority that you should eat what you are served. The laws of hospitality overrule any diet that does not involve the concept of sin. But here's what the Good Book has to say on the subject in Corinthians 10:27:

If one of the unbelievers invites you to dinner and you are disposed to go, eat whatever is set before you without raising any question on the ground of conscience.

If something will make you sick, don't eat it. But don't talk about it either. If it isn't on your cultist diet and you accepted a dinner invitation, don't turn this into an opportunity to give a lecture on why you are only eating gourds and spelt. Eat your dinner and shut up about it.

In this world of corporate sponsorship, being a guest is often a consequence of one's position in business rather than in society (and more and more those orders of pecking are one and the same), but you will still find yourself invited on occasion because you are liked. Being invited for your delightful personality is always more gratifying than being invited in the hope that you will write up the house for *Elle Decor* or testify for the defense at your host's next trial.

But no matter how desirable you are as a guest, you must participate effectively in conversation. Hopefully your wit, anecdotal richesse, and admirable aplomb will charm your companions and delight your host. Here are a few guidelines for conversation:

You were probably not invited for your skill as a debater. Everyone likes a lively discussion, but contention over dinner is a drag. Only people who are in absolute agreement should discuss religion at a friendly gathering. It should never, ever be discussed at a dinner party. As the wise H. L. Mencken noted:

We must respect the other fellow's religion…in the sense and to the extent that we respect his theory that his wife is beautiful and his children smart.

Politics have their place. It's called Congress. Avoid social discussion of the wretched affairs of state at all costs, at least until everyone is drunk enough that they won't remember what you said the next day. If you are in the company of intelligent people, don't act as if politics aren't important. But be clever and diplomatic. When prodded or cornered, use a perfect subject-changing line such as "Did you watch C-Span this afternoon?" Or "I think you need to look into what the Brookings Institution says." This will immediately signal to your opponent that there is no use trotting out the usual clichés because you can outbore them, and they will desist.

At dinner we are all friends, except, of course, with our most deadly enemies, and even then it shouldn't show. Hatred must hold its breath in the face of hospitable decorum. If you can't say anything nice, do it anyway. Andy Warhol's basic social strategy was to answer almost everything with "Gee, that's great!" When he said this in response to something glaringly awful, the offender would take him at his word while everyone else assumed he was kidding. Try it. It works. In this age of cutthroat maneuvering, you need all the friends you can get.

Overnight Guests

When you accept an invitation to stay at the home of another person, you are entering into an unspoken contract. The rules are unstated, but they are still there. You arrive when expected and depart on schedule. You do not show up with an unexpected date, sidekick, child, or pet. You do not show up empty-handed.

Bring good wines, amusing cordials, flowers, and chocolates, or if you are on the same taste wavelength, you may bring a gift for the house such as a candle or a whisk broom made by ancient Japanese methods. I had a guest arrive recently with an electric corkscrew that turned out to be a necessity of life.

Make your bed. Even if you don't make it at home.

Unless the house is staffed, offer to set the table and help clear it. Offer to do the dishes. Or dry. Pitch in without intruding. But if they tell you to sit down, take the hint.

If you sleep in the nude, do it at home. Pajamas should be worn in case of fire, medical emergency, robbery, or acts of God. Guests should also bring along a robe.

When occupying a guest room (as opposed to being the sole occupant of a guesthouse), do not cry out, shriek, or howl at orgasm, practice primal scream therapy, sob, blubber, or argue audibly with your spouse or date.

When you are a houseguest, the most important rule is, do not overstay your welcome—better to err on the side of leaving early. If it's too early, your hosts will beg you to stay for lunch.

Guests, whether for dinner or a weekend, should always write a thank-you note. E-mail shows you are not a complete barbarian. A note handwritten on stationery, sent by the U.S. mail, preferably with a nice commemorative stamp, shows that you really care.

HOW TO DINE OUT

One of life's great pleasures is dining out. As one gets older, it takes over the role of "nightlife." And while I certainly enjoyed taking in great bands in small clubs and getting up for the downstroke at famous discotheques, I would not trade in my restaurant life for that today. Matters of food and wine aside, I can't remember a great many conversations held in loud nightclubs, whereas shards of sparkling conversation from memorable dinners are still within recall.

While "foodies" rush about from this newly heralded restaurant to that one in search of the culinary grail, or the latest fashion in molecular gastronomy or recherché ethnic cuisine, I prefer being a regular in a few very good restaurants. Obviously one advantage is in the preferential treatment that inevitably attaches to consistent patronage. If the restaurant of your choice is often booked up, regular appearances will earn you the ability to secure the best table or last-minute seating when those opportunities would be unavailable to others. It is also impressive to one's guests when the owner, host, or waitstaff knows your name and is friendly to you and familiar with your preferences and habits. And sometimes, when the owner or management is feeling expansive or inebriated, the regular will be treated to an extra appetizer, dessert, or glass of wine. In short, the regular feels at home but better, utterly comfortable with no dishes to do.

I find the owners and operators of very good restaurants are often the kind of people I like. They value food, wine, and congenial people. A great restaurant cultivates good patrons and discourages the bad, boisterous loud talkers, indiscreet imbibers, and those with a distorted sense of entitlement. Of course, this sort will occasionally find its way into even the best establishments, but first-class operators find a way to get them out quickly and discourage their return. Fortunately bozo gourmands are conspicuous consumers and so they tend to favor restaurants that can compete with them in pretension.

The best restaurants generally have wonderful food and wine at prices that are fair but high enough to discourage bargain hunters or out-of-town adventurers. Thus the best restaurants approach the status of a club, being mostly devoted to a regular and loyal clientele.

In addition to a few favorite haunts, it's good to have alternative spots where you are known. Your familiarity can be expedited by generous tipping. Few funds are better spent than gratuities honoring good service. When one intends to become a regular or known at a restaurant, it is good to take one's time. It's better to be noticed for your attendance, good taste, and impeccable behavior than to call attention to yourself or attempt to get chummy with the staff.

We often see movie characters tipping headwaiters to get a table in a hot restaurant. In my experience, any place where this approach works is probably not worth patronizing. This is not to say that hosts and maîtres d's should never be tipped. They should be tipped during a holiday visit, on their birthday if you know it, or in the event that you throw a party in the place.

Reservations

Always give your full name, not just your last name, when making a reservation, both in case they have heard of you and so they will remember you better in the future.

If you're having trouble getting a reservation, call back and try prefacing your last name with "Congressman." Table for six for Congressman O'Brien? Of course! I've also noticed the names Auchincloss and Roosevelt work better than my own in certain jurisdictions.

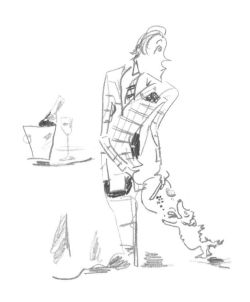

At the Table

Napkins should be placed on your lap when everyone is seated and not before. At lunch the napkin should be unfolded halfway, at dinner all the way. Don't ask me why, but I like this rule. Disregard it if lunch involves tomato sauce.

Restaurateurs please note: I would prefer to put my own napkin on my own lap. Also, I really don't need to know the name of the server, unless I wish to lodge a complaint later, in which case I will ask for it

Ordering for a lady may seem gallant, but it can also be obnoxious. If you have discussed the bill of fare extensively with the ladies in your party then you can order for them, if they would like that, but they may prefer to handle this adult chore solo. Just ask: "Shall I order?" Never order anything for anyone that they have not explicitly chosen themselves unless you know the food better than anyone and your party has given you carte blanche.

Ladies first. Host last.

Sending Back the Wine

You can't send a bottle back because you don't care for the wine, although if the sommelier suggests it he will likely volunteer to take it back. (And drink it himself later.) Properly, you can only send the wine back when it is corked, cooked, or otherwise spoiled. There shouldn't be any question about this because the wine is either bad or it isn't, and the sommelier or whoever performs that function should recognize this. You can usually peg a corked bottle from a single whiff of the wine. Also, if a bottle is bad the restaurant won't be stuck with it—they can return it to the distributor.

I remember once finding the proprietor of one of my haunts particularly inebriated one evening, after the *New York Times* had run a piece about how to return a bottle of wine. He had drunk several bottles just to prove the customer isn't always right.

The Tab

The person who invited the others should pick up the tab. It is, of course, sporting to challenge this. Very briefly. Don't argue over the check. It can get ugly as we try to one-up one another with largesse. If you really want to pick up the tab, arrange that beforehand or on your way to or from the men's room, but don't pull this maneuver if you have been invited to dinner.

It's fine for friends to split the check, but if one member of the party orders the Waverly Inn truffled macaroni and cheese for seventy-five dollars and drinks four Hennessy Paradis cognacs after dinner, he shouldn't suggest splitting the tab; he should pull out the credit card and suck it up like a man.

If you are splitting the tab and everyone tosses out plastic, toss out plastic; if everyone tosses cash, toss cash. A waiter is not an accountant. If your group hands over five credit cards, reflect this chore in the tip.

Tipping

Give the coat-check person a dollar per coat. Two dollars if they are attractive. Add a dollar for each hat, umbrella, and package.

I have very rarely stiffed a server, even a really bad one. If they have ruined your meal, give them ten percent. It's more insulting than nothing. If your server is horrible, complain to the boss. Adequate service gets fifteen percent; good service deserves twenty percent.

If the wine steward has taken care of the wine, tip the steward for the wine and the waiter for the rest of the tab.

If someone else in your party picks up the tab and then undertips, toss some makeup money down after the miserly host has left the crime scene. Fair is fair, and you may be back; why suffer guilt by association?

Incorrect Bills

It is certainly possible that a restaurant bill will contain errors. Waiting on tables is a high-pressure job, and good restaurants are often busy, increasing the potential for error. Many men consider adding up the bill déclassé. In fact, checking the bill is simply common sense. It's not all that unusual to get the tab from another table.

Over the years I have noticed that certain restaurants are more likely to make mistakes in the tab. This could mean that the waiter's job is particularly hectic here, but not if the mistakes invariably favor the house. The fix may be in. Don't be afraid to do the math and point out any mistakes you find—but if you find an error in your favor and don't alert the server, than you are no better than a bill-padding waitstaff. If you experience consistent mistakes in favor of the house, ask them for a copy of the detailed bill and open a file.

Sometimes there is an element of mystery in the billing process. The bill at a very chic Chinese restaurant I used to frequent never seemed to have a direct relation to what was ordered; it seemed more of a function of what kind of night they were having. But I never complained—well, maybe once or twice—because it seemed like an integral part of the experience. Some cultures bargain, some don't.

The most incorrect bill of all is the one delivered to the table that hasn't requested it yet.

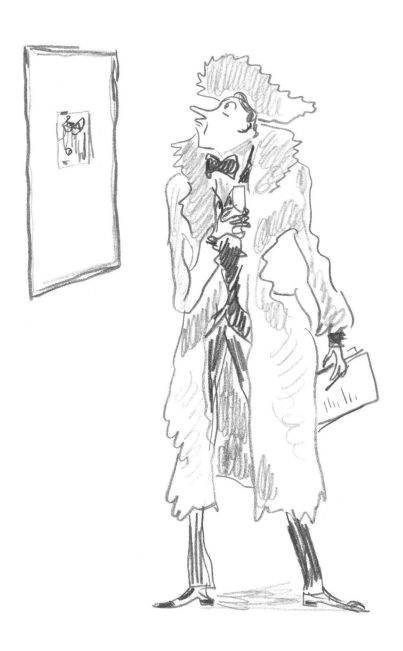

ON THE SNOB

"J'suis snob... Encore plus snob que tout à l'heure
Et quand je serai mort
J'veux un suaire de chez Dior!"

—Boris Vian, *Je Suis Snob*

According to the 13th Duke of Bedford, the first Peer of the Realm to open his estate to paying tourists, the term "snob" owes its origin to the medieval practice at Oxford and Cambridge of marking the names of commoner students with the words *sine nobilitate* ("without nobility"), which was eventually abbreviated to *s. nob.* Naturally the nontitled lads who found themselves competing socially with hereditary title heritors were inclined to try a little harder. They "out-peered the peers" is how Bedford puts it.

As cities grew up, industry, commerce, and colonization created that new breed, the middle class, which naturally began to strive for the finer things as developed by and exemplified in the manner of the royals. In fact, the new strivers strove to beat the royals at their own game, and since the royals were conditioned to think of striving as beneath their rank, the field was relatively unguarded.

William Makepeace Thackeray, author of *Vanity Fair*, among other satirical novels, wrote and illustrated *The Book of Snobs* (1848), a collection of essays that popularized the term. Thackeray observed that the more nobility depended on the wealth of exceptional commoners, the more opportunities the latter upstarts had to ascend to royal heights of glamour and obliterate the "sans" for themselves and their heirs. Thackeray put the reward of peerage deliciously:

"Your merits are so great," says the nation, "that your children shall be allowed to reign over us… It does not in the least matter that your eldest son be a fool: we think your services so remarkable that he shall have the reversion of your honours when death vacates your noble shoes."

We can imagine that there have been snobs as long as one man has bowed to another, but snobbism was a phenomenon of the nineteenth century because it wasn't until then that society could be climbed spectacularly by those without title. Beau Brummell, the commoner who was BFF status of the Prince Regent (later King George IV), was the first true celebrity. Brummell's extraordinary style and manner prompted the prince to embrace him as a confidant (if not idol), which elevated that uncommon commoner to the highest levels of society and made him the most imitated man of his day. Brummell set a criterion for snobs that endures to this day. He showed that taste and behavior alone were enough to propel a man to the heights and, in doing so, he proved that in an age of democracy, publicity was trump. He was a tragic figure, however, as those who took him to the top eventually brought him low. Famous for cutting those he considered beneath him, Brummell went too far when he remarked to a companion of the portly prince who had recently been cool to him, "Alvanley, who is your fat friend?"

Brummell's fatal flaw was believing he needed no one, while snobs are social beings by definition, ranked by the quality and quantity of their admirers. Snobs needed royalty, and royalty needed snobs. The royals needed wealth; the snobs needed glory. While the snob class at first represented the triumph of the urbane bourgeoisie over the landed gentry, the new crowd of achievers quickly became the aristocracy's safety net. In democracies, as long as there were enough upwardly mobile wealthy, nobility would be preserved as a goal, a model, and the ultimate accessory.

Even today, if it weren't for snobs, there would be no royal families and no class of international pretenders to phantom thrones, for snobbism is essentially the religion of class, and its sacraments are knighthood and peerage. Snobbism is pretense, and there's no pretender like that to a throne. Nothing in our time seems to more resemble heaven than the delightful lives of princes and princesses from countries that happily deposed their families, and no honor seems more coveted than the knighthood conferred on remarkable achievers such as Bono, Bill Gates, Akio Morita, Michael Caine, Plácido Domingo, and Elton John. To be addressed as "Sir," in that special way, is magical. Only sainthood can top this honor, and that, being posthumous, is not nearly as enjoyable.

Today's snob is not much different from the trailblazers of two centuries ago. The snob lives for affect. His or her being is utterly contingent on the perceptions of others, and so the life of a snob is a continual effort to keep up appearances and manipulate the social milieu in hope of salvation through publicity, while holding others to the same standards of judgment. The snob may be a flatterer and a toady, but a study of nature reveals that evolution favors the flatterer as much as it does the warrior, and flattery is far easier and safer than combat.

In the twentieth century, money largely replaced land and title as the arbiter of class, but wealth is not enough, nor is fame. The snob recognizes and despises the traits of the newly wealthy and tends to behave as if he is so accustomed to wealth that he's above it; that his money is not the fruit of his considerable efforts, but was rather inconveniently foisted upon him by previous generations. It is OK to be suddenly rich, but it's not OK to behave that way. You don't want to be a nouveau riche parvenu. Of course, if you are a celebrity you are granted a certain immunity. The excesses of entertainers are tolerated with bemusement, but only so far. Note that Mick Jagger, Eric Clapton, and Jay-Z tend to wear the right sort of clothes and live in the right sort of home and cultivate relationships with the right sort of company. Snobbism forgives how you got there as long as once there, you play by the rules. It seems unlikely that Keith Richards will be knighted, or if he were, that he would accept. Although there are precedents, I suppose, like Sir Francis Drake and Sir Henry Morgan.

Passing judgment is the snob's preoccupation. Everything is critiqued and ruled upon. You are judged by your education, your occupation, your address, the decor of your home, the art and books found there, your clothing, jewelry, and deportment. You will also be judged by your children's school, where you vacation, your automobile, and the stores and services you patronize. There are safety zones, however—as you will not generally be judged by your knowledge or ideas. Your flaws will not be attacked as long as they are consistent with those of your peers, and certain forms of folly are encouraged, such as treating small dogs like spoiled children.

Snobbism is not a characteristic of a particular class. Servants are often greater snobs than their employers, and there are few snobs of greater snobbiness than the help in luxury-brand boutiques—who seem determined to impress the customer with their total disdain—or the maître d's and waiters in smart restaurants. In Paris recently, I was greatly amused by a waiter at Fouquet's. When I asked if they had Coca-Cola, he paused and said derisively, "Yes, but it is no good!" Perhaps you remember Bijan, the large, pricey Fifth Avenue store where a doorman judged whether or not you were worthy of admittance? Or the trouble Oprah had getting in the door of Hermès in Paris? And you have certainly noticed overdressed boutique salespeople chatting on and on idly while you're helping yourself. There's no snob like a shop clerk unless it's a doorman. And buzzers and velvet ropes and VIP rooms continue to spread across cities as the unimportant hope that making a show of keeping people out will be enough to make them want in.

The snob's interest in you is directly proportional to the sum of the grandeur in the room. He may appear to be among your best friends at a small cocktail gathering, but he will cut you quite dead at the Met's Costume Institute Gala. The snob is always tentative, ready to adjust and temper his responses according to ephemeral shifts in apparent social position.

The snob invariably refers to celebrities by first name only: "And then Marlon called... I was talking with Gwyneth..." That is, unless the name like George or Johnny is insufficient to register precisely, whereupon, after a petulant pause, he may clarify, appending a surname: Clooney, Depp, etc.

There are snob ideals. Snobs value charity greatly; in fact, it is almost compulsory. But money is not to be given quietly. It must be given at a grand party, often in exchange for art donated by hardworking painters who don't even get a tax deduction for it.

Snobs often avoid political discussion, not because they have no thoughts on the matter, but because of the extreme difficulty of pulling off an opinion without offering offense. So the successful snob lets his actions speak for him, championing the environment by driving a hybrid bumper stickered with "Riverkeeper," "Free Tibet," and, if he's daring, "Greenpeace," and attempting to push the co-op board to switch to fluorescent bulbs in public places. Intelligent snobs are beginning to discuss their personal carbon footprint and are trying to figure out how to write some of it off to their business or entourage. Environmentalism is very chic, and an extremely rich field for the snob hobbyist. While horses are still tops, it is increasingly admired to have herds of sheep and goats and make your own artisanal cheese, or even to raise breeds of cattle seldom seen outside the Channel Islands. Or to grow ramps, Treviso, and heirloom tomatoes, or open a biodynamic vineyard. Americans are discovering what Brits have known for generations: posing as a farmer, especially an organic farmer, is golden.

Most of the old techniques of snobbism discussed by Thorstein

Veblen in *The Theory of the Leisure Class* still hold, although they have evolved. Conspicuous consumption has become codified consumption, and conspicuous waste, being nongreen, is indulged mostly in the guise of entertaining friends or performing acts of charity. Whereas once you might have flown a jumbo jet full of friends to Marrakech for a blowout, today you do it to benefit a group of sufferers, the more pathetic the better. Fashion is still crucial, especially for the female snob, and while environmentalism has its prominent place, one still does not wear last year's collection. The true environmentalist puts the hopelessly "last year" items away until they are "vintage," or he donates them to charity for a fat tax write-off.

Uselessness was long a benchmark of wealth, and anything smacking of utility and practicality was seen as hopelessly vulgar, but in recent decades a confluence of factors has led to something of a revolution. Old fashion was a mark of wealth because one could obviously not perform manual labor or even move without assistance while so attired. Today, however, society has gone casual for two reasons. First, in a postindustrial age, there are legions of vulgar and impecunious persons who also do little manual labor, so the rejection of practical attire has lost its former meaning. Second, the wealthy class requires camouflage. There are at least eight million millionaires in the United States and more than 400 billionaires. (Time to bring back society's 400?) The top one percent possesses nearly fifty percent of all the wealth. Obviously there is increased resentment, even though the have-nots seem to consistently vote for policies advantageous to the have-lots, partially because of political bait-and-switch tactics, and partially because in America the poor tend to believe that they can and will become rich. They vote for billionaire tax relief in the same reckless spirit of optimism in which they purchase lotto tickets. "Casual Fridays" and the increasingly prevalent casual office helps prevent the rich from standing out and the poor from feeling denied. Fortunately, fashion is resilient and designers have been able to create clothing that can only be recognized as expensive by the class that wears it, so that the wealthy can recognize one another while remaining fairly inconspicuous to the hoi polloi. Jeans and sneakers push four figures while limited editions are the rage in shoes, handbags, belts, and tees. We are seeing the emergence of a Freemasonry of fashion, a mode in code.

Snobbism is a race, a competition. It's about getting there first and leaving first: being the first to patronize a new restaurant and the first to abandon it when, as Yogi Berra said, "It's so crowded nobody goes there anymore." Snobs complain about this constant displacement, even though it is of their own doing. The people who moan the most about the crowds in the Hamptons and St. Barts and at the Waverly Inn are the last ones into the place.

It's not easy being a snob. Fashions change so quickly that the snob must be hypervigilant, ready to jump off the bandwagon at precisely the right moment, leaving friends and even family behind to remain "on the tip." The snob is always doing a balancing act between apparent virtue and actual cruelty—but of course nature is cruel, so he can write off the victims of his slights and the friends he left behind to "survival of the fittest." The snob must be prepared to employ strange posturing tactics, sometimes called reverse snobbery, as soon as he feels crowded. There is no radical like the aristocrat. Luchino Visconti, the Duke of Madrone, saw no contrariety in belonging to the Italian Communist Party. The snob exists beyond irony.

To succeed the snob must continually make judgments, apparently on principle but informed by whimsicality. The essential irony of the snob was best expressed by Groucho Marx: "I wouldn't join any club that would have me as a member." For the snob it's all about the newest information, the latest development, and the struggle to be in early and on the money can be brutal. As Elaine de Kooning said, "Frank [O'Hara] says nobody looks at dead artists anymore. Living artists have become snobs about being alive."

We're all snobs, one way or another. The good snob is the one who uses his upward mobility to improve himself, to develop real character, and to graduate and lose that *"sine"* and become *"nobilitate."* Since nobility is extinct, we have to reinvent it. We have to nobilitate ourselves. In the end, being a snob is its own reward and/or punishment. The snobs who achieve transcendence are a lucky few. But when we do, we generally recognize one another. Depending, of course, on who else is in the room.

HOW TO BE POLITE

Yes, Virginia, civilization did end. But in case it comes back, we don't want to be left out, do we? In the meantime, behaving with style and aplomb will both impress those we want as friends and frighten our enemies. Exemplary behavior will make sure the welcome mat is always out when we visit and that the answering machine won't pick up when we call. Here are a few basic considerations on behavior in an anything-goes world.

• Always acknowledge the people you know. Success in society—or what passes for it—only comes to those with good communication skills. Some people have the terrible habit of gravitating only to those they perceive as their betters—I'm sure you know people who say "hi" to you when there are ten people in the room but ignore you when there are fifty. You should greet people you know even when you can't remember their name. This is a democracy and even if they aren't in a position to give you money, they may have a chance to get back at you. Nice up! If you can't remember her name, just tell her how fabulous she looks that will give you time to figure it out.

• Don't automatically introduce people. Unless you're sure it's a good idea, don't. Everyone doesn't have to know everyone. Some people already hate one another without your knowledge or help.

- Don't hide your mistakes; they may be the best part of your résumé. Since the mid-eighties, we have lived in a culture of recovery. I think it's something we picked up from the space program. By the nineties, chic twelve-step meetings surpassed the country club and the VIP room as the place to shine. Everyone has a few skeletons in the closet. They make your profile spicier and provide real contrast: "Oh, he's wonderful now. He used to be such a mess." If you were awful enough, you might even get a book out of it. But learn from Oprah: slug it "fiction."

- Don't flaunt your wealth. Obviousness is so obvious. Let others figure out just how rich you are, and they'll enjoy you so much more. If you keep reminding them of your success, they may soon tire of you. When it comes to costs—don't ask, don't tell. Fortunately, we live in a clever age where it's possible to find clothes that look like poor people's clothes. No one will mug you on the street, but those in the know will recognize that those torn, abraded, and perfectly soiled jeans have a four-figure price tag. There is nothing morally wrong with a Maybach, but you will get more mileage with a Prius. All the really rich people are driving them, and they position you as an idealist who can afford to be. Subtle cheapness is the sign of real wealth.

- Be cool with the help. Nothing is more of a turnoff than someone who is rude to waiters, hotel housekeeping, drivers, salespeople, and the like. I once dropped a former Miss Universe contestant for being snotty to waiters. I remember, after a recent economic downturn, seeing a former investment whiz selling suits in a well-known store. He should have been nicer when he was on top. That old one about being nice to people on the way up because you'll meet them on the way down…what if it's true? And who do you think plants all those gossip-page items about egoists behaving badly?

- Spread gossip selectively. If you want to get good stuff, you have to be as discreet as a secret society. If you say you won't tell, don't. Test people by telling them and only them a story, possibly fictional, and swear them to secrecy. Then see if it gets back to you.

• Wait until they mention it. Reserve commenting on their pregnancy, facelift, or liposuction until they bring it up first. Sometimes the light plays tricks on us. Same thing with the divorce or the lawsuit. Sometimes our information is wrong. Never take sides in a divorce until it is final. And even then don't.

• In the event that name-dropping is required, do it right. Use the last name too and you won't sound quite so ridiculous. Quentin, Jude, Jack, Kirsten, Gwyneth…don't make me guess. You're enough work already.

• Don't tell people they are dressed wrong. You might think you are helping someone who is a mess, and maybe you are, but at the risk of being hated. Think of it this way: dressed as they are now, they make you look even better. Without the tacky, the unsightly, and the fashion victimized, there would be no best-dressed list.

• Always say thank you. Say it even when you're not grateful. Even when you're angry. You'll get them thinking and worrying: "Was he serious? Have I gone too far this time? What's he up to?" Kill them with cordiality. Write notes. Send e-mails. Put "thank you" down on paper. But be careful about "I love you." Magnanimity is rare and magnificent. Thank you for reading this.

HOW TO BE AN INDIVIDUAL

It's not easy to be yourself, but really you have no other choice. It seems like everything has been done and everything has been said. You're a guy—just another guy. There are probably dozens of people out there with your name. Personally, I share a name with a motorcycle racer, a heavy metal musician, a real estate broker, and an easy-listening DJ who writes a blog—and those are just the sort-of-famous ones. A few years ago, another blogger wrote how sad it was that I ended up an easy-listening DJ.

But that's the way it goes in a world of billions. You feel like a replicant, a molecule. Facebook says, "Not the John Doe you were looking for?" And the world has become so modular that existence demands that you fit in somewhere. Where's a man without a slot, a role, a position? Which usually means altering yourself to fit your place. As some cat once said, "To go with the flow is a cold crush."

Once men were unique simply because they were; today we feel pressure to alter ourselves just so we won't be like everybody else. You've got no clan, no tribe, no fraternity to help you. You're on your own, on your own recognizance, and you don't know who you are. You want to rebel, but rebellion itself has become so typical and conformist that it's just a more desperate pose. A generation or two ago, it was easy to find the outsiders—they stood out. They might have a tattoo, or a piercing, or dress in a weird, nonconformist way, but today's fashion followers and even mainstream youth have adopted the appearances of yesterday's freaks, outcasts, and eccentrics, making it difficult to tell the normals from the deviants without a program.

In the fifties and sixties, if you encountered significant tattoos, long hair, facial hair, and piercings, someone attired in leathers, a dashiki, or a frock coat, chances are you were dealing with a genuine freak—a psychopath or sociopath, a druggy or criminal perhaps, an anarchist, a junkie, or a self-taught shaman, someone with a scheme or a plot, an agenda or a tendency.

Today we see people who look exactly like those old-time partisans of extravagance, but these dangerously styled and provocatively appointed persons are replicas and facsimiles of the rebels of the past. They got their personality out of a catalog. You could say that they are fakes, but I think you would be wrong because we live in an age that has outlived authenticity itself. Everything is a simulation. "Realness" is just another category at the voguing ball.

To understand how we came to this pass, let's consider freak history. When I was a wild youth, "freak" was a term in derisive use, but we adopted it as a compliment. Alternative folks circa the Summer of Love didn't call themselves hippies or flower children. That would have been embarrassing. We called ourselves freaks the way gays later took to calling themselves queer, turning the slur into a proclamation of pride.

We were freaks because our looks were deliberately aberrant. In his coolly ominous, bluesy "If 6 Was 9," Jimi Hendrix, perhaps the most flagrantly freaky man on the planet, sang about the "white-collar conservatives...pointing their plastic finger at me," declaring, "I'm gonna wave my freak flag high." We were the flags, the standards of our own movement, each one slightly different. The freaks were a spiritual fraternity, demarcated from the mass by clear visual evidence: long hair, beards, and costumes that bespoke a more particular and committed role than did normal civil attire.

The word "freak" comes from the Old English *frician*, meaning "to dance"; in its oldest sense, it means "a capricious humor, notion, whim, or vagary." Only later did it come to mean an aberration or monstrosity, as in a freak show. Tod Browning's 1932 feature film *Freaks* explored that world of human oddities, with a cast including pinheads, midgets, Siamese twins, basket cases, a hermaphrodite, and "the living torso." And to the stoned freaks of the sixties, those natural freaks, those mutants who had no choice in the matter, provided a model of camaraderie for the volunteer freaks who were emerging as a mass movement, creating deliberate mutations in art, music, politics, sexuality, and consciousness itself.

"To freak out" originally meant to react badly to drugs you had taken; eventually, it denoted any sort of extreme behavior resembling chemically induced antics. To freak out was to "wig out" or "blow your mind." In an atmosphere where strangeness earned a certain respect, "freak out" began to take on a positive spin. By 1981, when Chic released the hit disco song "Le Freak," the refrain "freak out" had redeemed the word "freak" and taken it right back to its roots in dance. Today one is likely to hear "Get your freak on," referring to dancing or something similar that's done in a prone position.

Society has always had freak subcultures of one sort or another, from the dandies of the Restoration and the bohemians of the nineteenth century to the beatniks of the fifties, hippies of the sixties, punks of the seventies, and goths of the eighties. But the freak mode seemed to accelerate as the bohemian became both the avant-garde and a notion tied to time, progress, and yes, fashion.

In the sixties, Marshall McLuhan, the first philosopher of pop, explained the changes going down in his book *The Medium is the Massage*, in which he said that technology had shrunk the planet into a global village, spawning a new tribalism. The hippies were tribal, assembling into affinity groups and drawing inspiration from pioneers, mountain men, sadhus, sorcerers, Victorians, Native Americans, cowboys, pirates, pagans, and other roles that resonated in their acid-fueled imaginations.

There's a wonderful description of hippies in Norman Mailer's *Armies of the Night*, a 1968 account of the 1967 peace march on the Pentagon:

The hippies were there in great number...dressed like the legions of Sgt. Pepper's Band, some were gotten up like Arab sheiks, or in Park Avenue doormen's greatcoats, others like Rogers and Clark of the West, Wyatt Earp, Kit Carson, Daniel Boone in buckskin...and wild Indians with feathers, a hippie gotten up like Batman, another like Claude Rains in *The Invisible Man*—his face wrapped in a turban of bandages and he wore a black satin top hat. They were close to being assembled from all the intersections between history and the comic books, between legend and television, the Biblical archetypes and the movies.

Mailer sensed that this costumed horde represented something quite new, and that it had been conjured out of an electrochemically linked-up collective unconscious through the agency of LSD and rock music. In his words, "the history of the past was being exploded right into the present." Mailer understood that the hippie was not merely costumed for battle but costumed for a transformed life. The hippie appeared as a channeled character, as something "other" dredged up from a shared fantasy of history.

Mailer wrote:

If nature was a veil whose tissue had been ripped by static, screams of jet motors, the highway grid of the suburbs, smog, defoliation, pollution of streams, overfertilization of the earth, anti-fertilization of women, and the radiation of two decades of near blind atom busting, then perhaps the history of the past was another tissue, spiritual, no doubt...nonetheless being bombed by the use of LSD as outrageously as the atoll of Eniwetok, Hiroshima, Nagasaki, and the scorched foliage of Vietnam.

Mailer saw the freaks as fallout from LSD's atom-smashing of consciousness. But what he witnessed among the hippie hordes wasn't necessarily an unconscious acting out of some chromosome-stored film loop of a past life, being spooled out on the cutting room floor of history. It was a conscious rejection of the future as planned by its partisans.

As Arthur Rimbaud wrote: "Le monde marche! Pouquoi ne tournera it il pas?" Time marches on! Why not about-face? The freaks saw the future and decided they weren't going there. They were going back. The freaks would beam themselves back into a historical mentality and cultural mode more to their liking, doing their own thing among like-minded free spirits. But the unstructured hippies could only float along, dreaming of another way. Some went communal, organic, and alternative, but many just went to the barbershop then the office.

In the documentary film *The Filth and the Fury,* Malcolm McLaren comments sadly on the fact that punk began as a form of extreme individualism and soon turned into just another stereotype. Today I see full-on teen punks who look like space aliens who saw *Summer of Sam* from ten light-years away and thought the Mohawk was normal. I can only assume that like hippies of the acid days, they are trying to dream up a world they feel passed them by but which never really existed. In New York, punk style happened long after punk rock, created by people imitating a rumor.

There hasn't been a spontaneous mass display of originality in years. And yet there are still freaks out there, genuine freaks. Most of the true freaks I see now are women, often wealthy women, over the age of seventy. They are the most completely artificial of creatures because little remains of what nature gave them. They are human artifacts, self-made works of art (despite their reliance on the arts of the surgeon, the designer, and the hairdresser). The real freak is an original, not a copy. Freak movements will come and go, but the true freak is always a solo act, struggling determinedly against the easy way out.

Being an individual is lonely. And in our world of titanic corporations, monolithic states, and mind-control media, absolutist conformity is strictly enforced. It seems that only the self-employed can be self-styled and original. Even then it's difficult. As soon as someone manages to break out of the mold, he is imitated, cloned, and marketed, and pretty soon there's a new mold. I wonder if any sort of mobilized mass eccentricity is still possible. I admit I am nostalgic for freak solidarity and the power it promised, and I await some meaningful badge by which I can pledge my allegiance to otherness. No Mohawks, please. "MWM looking for like-minded adult eccentrics..."

In a 1958 article for *Esquire*,[1] Jack Kerouac wrote:

The Beat Generation. That was a vision that we had, John Clellon Holmes and I, and Allen Ginsberg in an even wilder way, the late forties of a generation of crazy, illuminated hipsters suddenly rising and roaming America, serious bumming and hitchhiking everywhere, ragged, beatific, beautiful in an ugly graceful new way—a vision gleaned from the way we had heard the word "beat" spoken on street corners on Times Square and in the Village, in other cities in the downtown-city-night of postwar America—"beat" meaning down and out but full of intense conviction.

The funny thing about our time is that it is all times, all eras at once. It's sort of time squared. Walk down the street and you still see the beats, or reasonable facsimiles thereof. You see hippies and punks and piratical Jack Sparrow dandies. If you can dress it, it exists. Lots of people feel out of synch with this time, so they choose their own ideal era, but they aren't the only ones with that taste in a particular cultural time, and so there are communities of alternative time out there—little islands of history floating in the present.

Maybe the solution is to get outside the mainspring of the time machine, culturally reincarnating into the past. I think we need to revive the old jobs—shepherd, stonemason, thatcher, goatherd, poet—and the old practices like quilting bees, contract bridge, and yodeling, before we disappear down the Internet rabbit hole into digital limbo. Some days I feel like I can see a new, older future walking down the street.

I remember when Marshall McLuhan's pop philosophy was new and how great it was to think of the miniskirt as a tribal costume. Woodstock was called a gathering of the tribes, but we had no idea what we were doing. We couldn't pull off a revolution. But today there's more room to maneuver. We have all of cyberspace to navigate, and we've got better tools to locate our proper tribes. The more we cultivate our individual otherness, the sooner we will find enough like-minded oddballs to form cool contemporary tribes for fun and profit.

---

1   Jack Kerouac, "Aftermath: The Philosophy of the Beat Generation," *Esquire*, March 1958.

HOW TO BE A FRIEND

Don't you hate it when a perfectly good word changes its meaning? Like "friend"? It's so confusing. Now we've got to start all over.

What is a friend today in the age of Facebook? What does friendship entail in the digital demimonde? Where do you draw the line between friend and acquaintance in a world where people "friend" those with whom they are not even acquainted? What is the difference between a friend and a contact? Between a friend, a Roman, and a countryman? Is friendship with women possible? I'll tell you what I'd tell a friend.

Ideally a friend is someone you have actually met, someone you like and spend time with, although it is possible to establish a friendship through diligent correspondence, particularly if one party is incarcerated. Traditionally, friendship required time; it demanded a certain intimacy that was not granted instantly. Today, however, thanks to the digital exploitation of common personal weaknesses, it is now widely believed that it is possible for one's résumé or curriculum vitae to become friends with other people's résumés or curricula vitae.

A friend is defined as a person whom one knows, likes, and trusts. A person, not a set of data. "Friend" is a noun, and its use as a transitive verb is unfortunate and hopefully a fad. I do not wish to friend or be friended, although I don't mind the occasional befriending. One thing that bothers me about "friend" as a verb is that friendship is a mutual state, whereas "friending" someone is a unilateral action. It's aggressive, more like stalking than embracing.

I get lots of requests to be friends from people I don't know because I do happen to be listed on MySpace and Facebook. An actual friend of mine made me a MySpace page and I have about 350 "friends" there, although only fifteen or so are people I actually know—the rest are mostly young musicians, because this network is a place where kids can post music. But you do wind up with odd "friends" who aren't even acquaintances. I got a request from Ondine, the Warhol superstar, whom I actually knew, and his profile says that he's seventy-three. In fact, he died in 1989. I also seem to be friends with Frida Kahlo and I have no memory of that friendship, but she has been dead since I was seven.

I put myself on Facebook because my son was living in Korea and I heard he was posting a lot of photos that he forgot to e-mail me, so I joined under an assumed name. Oddly, people figured out it is me, so now people I don't know want to be my assumed identity's friend on Facebook.

Hardly a week passes that I don't get an e-mail saying that someone wants to add me to his or her professional network on LinkedIn. And usually the person who wants to "link me in" is someone I have minimal and completely sufficient links with. I don't want to be LinkedIn. I want to be LinkedOut.

Friendships are sometimes spoken of as Platonic, usually by people who have never read Plato. By this is meant a relationship that does not involve eroticism, and therefore "Platonic" is often used as a dismissal of intention in relationships where a physical aspect might prove socially prob-lematic—such as between those married to others. The *Oxford English Dictionary* defines "Platonic" as "applied to love that is purely spiritual for one of the opposite sex. (As originally used, *amor platonicus* was a synonym of *amor socraticus*, denoting the kind of interest in young men with which Socrates was credited, and had no reference to women.)" Maybe it's time we went back to include the original meaning of "Platonic." It sounds a lot better than "man crush" or "bromance." Mutual-admiration society anyone? As for nonsexual relationships with the opposite sex, we could just say, "We have a non-fucking relationship."

As the digital landscape of social networks grows, Twittering minute by minute toward some critical mass, people make assumptions about strangers that seem destined to result in disappointment, much as dating services and other artificial communities did in the past. The wise man reserves his friendship for those who have proved worthy of it. Friendship is about quality, not quantity.

It is best to avoid any situation that offers "networking" as a benefit. Networking seems to mean "socializing with intent." This inelegant practice undoubtedly requires lowering one's guard, if not one's standards. The idea of mingling with a crowd of strangers in the hope of making "contacts" or even friends is a dismal one. It's best to take a romantic, fatalistic attitude toward friends or even contacts. If you are meant to be friends, it will happen. If you are meant to do business, it will be done. I believe friendship is fate; it is written. Inshallah! Soliciting friends only invites trouble.

There are various levels of friendship, and as people now term persons they do not even know as friends, it's time to be more specific about what we mean by the word. Someone we are linked to on a social network is not a friend but a digital acquaintance. Someone whom we have met but with whom we have not formed a bond of trust or reliance is an acquaintance. A friend is someone with whom we enjoy mutual admiration, easy access, and a certain degree of intimacy, confidence, and trust.

Society may not be as sexually promiscuous as it once was, but it is far more socially promiscuous. This is an age of "identity theft," but it is also an age of commerce posing as society. We are continually accosted, importuned, solicited, prevailed upon, and aggressively propositioned. Perfect strangers loud-hail us or track us down, setting up social ambushes and roadblocks to buttonhole us. Perfect strangers tutoyer us or attempt to perpetrate socialite air-kisses near our faces. Meaningless sentiments couched in intimate terms are transmitted randomly through impersonal networks.

Do not be afraid to notify inappropriate parties that they are out of bounds and over the line. Tell them they are not your friends and it is unlikely they ever will be your friends. Tell them that you do not accept solicitations or telephone calls from strangers, that they are not to contact you ever again, and if they do measures will be taken. A faux friend is a foe.

Socratic considerations aside, there are those who think that men and women cannot be friends. While this may be true in some cases, there is no reason why a man can't be friends with a woman. Among the evolved, it's a snap; however, adding sex to any friendship—whether hetero or homo—is bound to change the equation and the chemistry of the relationship. Proceed with caution, as men and women may have considerably different views on friendship's boundaries. It's prudent, generally, to avoid fucking your friends. A good friend is hard to find.

HOW TO FLY

I flew the Concorde with the greats. The passing of that elegant machine seemed to mark a permanent turn for the worse, not only in travel but also in the history of modernism itself, hence culture. I have flown first class, business class, premium economy, and economy. I have flown economy (once called coach) in conditions that would probably compare unfavorably with steerage class on the *Titanic*.

When I was a boy, flying was wonderfully luxurious adventure. It was almost a miracle to ascend into the sky in a beautiful, plushly decorated masterpiece of engineering, to see the world as the gods do and be served like royalty, and to arrive in an hour at a destination that would have otherwise required eight hours on the seemingly infinite Pennsylvania Turnpike, even then a congested antique scarier than *Ice Road Truckers*. (Well, *Ice Road Truckers* wasn't on yet, but there were ice-road truckers.)

On airliners, one traveled with the elite. Men in suits, women in pretty dresses. People actually dressed up to fly, perhaps, in part, because they wanted to impress the crew. Stewardesses (today known as flight attendants) were selected for their beauty and charm, while pilots were notoriously wealthy, pulling down salaries comparable to big-league ballplayers'.

It's almost painful now to remember those halcyon days, living as we are in a mass-transit national security state. Today, only premium classes approach what flying once was, and that's after you get to the airport and through security. In the class euphemistically referred to as economy, one is seated among persons one would ordinarily cross the street to avoid. Often fellow passengers, even female fellows, are obese and, strapped in with their seat-belt extensions, hanging over into your space. Gods forbid they should fall asleep, and on long flights they probably will pass out after consuming pharmaceuticals that transform them into sleep-eating Ambien zombies.

Food, if it is served, is fodder. Flight attendants are no longer like hosts and hostesses, stewards and maître d's, or hospitable caregivers; they are now a sort of a civilian branch of law enforcement—embittered disciplinarians and clerks, or on some airlines, failed stand-up comics.

These days I often find myself thinking, Do I *really* want to go? Frequently as a writer I am offered free trips to places I would really like to visit—just recently there was a golf junket to Morocco with first-class hotel accommodations. I still feel like a snob asking if the ticket is business class, but this has practically become a matter of life and death. I will plead back troubles, whatever it takes, but if that's the ticket I just won't go. Why? I want to return alive and well.

Travel today is not for amateurs. Amateurs are the ones holding up the line at the security checkpoint. To travel well now, we must be highly disciplined and observe strict tactical rules.

Rule number one: Do not fly economy on any trip that takes more than two hours. You will be treated as freight, although freight generally cannot be insulted. The law of the jungle informs every decision made in the back of the plane, as opposed to in business or first class. The front of the plane is air travel as it was intended (the police state aside). The back of the plane is about survival of the fittest, and what got us this far as a species may yet get us to Pittsburgh.

If you are a business traveler, your company should send you business class, obviously. If their new bare-bones policy restricts this, inform them of your lumbago, sciatica, restless leg syndrome, and, if necessary, your limited continence, claustrophobia, and panic attacks. Or figure out how to use your miles or someone else's or upgrade using the airline's plutonium card. Should you absolutely have no choice but to fly in economy, you must do whatever it takes to procure a bulkhead seat (inform them of your spontaneous projectile vomiting) or an exit row (of course you are willing to assist in an emergency, but don't look too happy about it). Some airlines now offer these slightly more humane seats at a premium; pay it.

Because of the heightened sense of security and insecurity on aircraft, I believe that midair is one place where ratting out one's fellow man is not only permissible but prudent. I'm not talking about fingering innocent Arabic speakers pointing at Mount Rushmore; I'm talking about guarding against airborne alcoholic blackouts and sedative bad trips. If the person next to you is behaving in a loutish, offensive, or possibly harmful manner, go to the stews. Make them deal with it. If the passenger next to you is too large for the seat, do not allow intrusion into your space or they will become Germany and you Poland. Complain. Push the little button with the human figure on it and turn on the charm.

If you drink, do so like a gentleman. Although it is unlikely to conform with airline policy, discreet flask use is certainly not rude or offensive but rather medicinal. The economy "bar" is unlikely to stock single malt or Armagnac. If you are caught, tell the flight attendant, "It's a prescription. It calms me."

While the seating, service, and amenities on today's airlines make unconsciousness a desirable state during flight, there are numerous downsides to this option. Should the plane go down, escape becomes a priority and in that case lucidity as well as nimbleness are desirable. The odds against a crash are, of course, astronomical, but when one is penned like an animal it's hard to avoid negative thoughts. (A word of warning, however: thinking that if one sleeps then the plane will crash is an early warning sign of delusional, solipsistic paranoia. If one sleeps the plane will not crash; if one perishes the world will not cease to exist.) Follow the advice of the flight attendant and remember where the closest exit is, and also consider whom you will have to fight and disable on your way there.

The same good-sense policy applies to drugs. Ambien zombies have ceased to be gentlemen. This widely prescribed drug is known to send people out onto the highways eating ice cream behind the wheel while believing they are abed asleep. It is quite likely that the fellow attempting to enter the cockpit or defecate on the service trolley is not in his usual mind and is under the influence of a prescription drug recommended by his personal physician, who is receiving kickbacks from a major pharmaceutical company. A gentleman is not carried off the plane except for natural causes, and stretchers and straitjackets are a must to avoid. I find that several glasses of good Bordeaux are usually enough to send me into an actual REM state for the transatlantic duration. If they aren't, I might nibble on a small-dose Valium tablet, never taking more than is necessary so as to avoid grogginess in Paris.

I recently watched *The High and the Mighty* (1954) and was greatly amused by its portrayal of midcentury airline travel. Not only was everyone smoking up a storm (and praying up a storm), but they were all dressed to the nines. Yes, that's the way it was—smart business attire. Today it's generally all about gym clothes on planes, the ba-da-bing tracksuit being what American men wear to fly, not just because of the vulgarization of society but also because air travel has become more physically demanding. I try to dress in as civil a manner as possible while allowing for the contortions that may be required in crawling over sleeping people. Polo shirts and knits travel better than broadcloth. Trousers with some stretch in the fabric may help prevent transatlantic crotch tingle or foot dozing. I always wear comfy slip-on shoes so that if I arrive at Heathrow with size fourteen feet instead of the usual twelve, I won't have to deplane barefoot.

Security

Arrive at the airport with a strap-on walking boot cast, so much more convenient than crutches. Get a wheelchair at curbside and be whisked to the head of the security line and straight to the gate. I experienced this extraordinary boon shortly after September 11, when I broke an ankle in the midst of a heavy travel schedule.

I have often thought of taking up the practice again. Is it cheating? I don't believe it is, as most of the occupants of wheelchairs are not actually disabled in the conventional sense but are too fat or old to walk. If airline officials question your need for a wheelchair, tell them you are old, fat, tired, or you have Epstein-Barr or depression. You have lost the will to walk. Call them motherfuckers and then tell them you have Tourette's syndrome.

I was reminded of this tactic recently when returning from the delightful island of Jamaica, from Montego Bay, a truly disastrous airport. The line for security snaked through the entire airport and looked to require a few hours for complete transit; meanwhile, Jamaicans, who apparently failed to absorb during the colonial era the British enthusiasm for queuing, began inserting themselves well up the line at places "saved" for them.

It was then that I noticed the fellow in a baseball cap bearing the logo of the Defense Intelligence Agency (which shows the Earth with a torch as its axis), with whom I had struck up a conversation in the check-in line. He had had golf clubs with him, and we had chatted about Jamaican courses we had played before he walked briskly up to the ticket agent. Now he was being pushed to the head of the security line in a wheelchair, his body language saying "disabled." He must have given the attendant ten U.S. dollars. He waved as he glided past on his way to the gate. That's why they call it "Intelligence."

You must also get yourself a FlyClear pass from the TSA, or make sure you have a ticket that entitles you to fast-track along with the first-class passengers and crew.

What else? Well, profiling by security is of course forbidden, but after being randomly searched a few times in a row, I have decided to trim my short beard down to mere stubble before heading to the airport.

Food Onboard

Airline food today is usually execrable except in upper classes on certain airlines. Even when traveling business, it's wise to eat first or bring along a tasty snack for a long flight in case they run out of something you will eat. Some airlines will not carry enough of each selection to serve the entire business cabin, so if they start serving in the wrong place you are likely to be stuck with the vegan headcheese soufflé.

In coach, you're a fool *not* to pack a meal. Kennels have better food than most airlines' economy class—and now you may have to pay for the slop too. Just don't bring something messy and smelly that will offend me if I'm sitting next to you. Hold the onions, hold the garlic, and don't even think about runny Gallic raw-milk cheeses.

Even economy class can be improved with a foie gras sandwich, a small jar of osetra, and a preboarding-administered opium suppository.

Airborne Distress

Generally the person over 300 pounds gets the "shared" armrest. Among equals, it's a toss-up and should be shared informally. Readers have more of a right than movie watchers. If the person in the business-class aisle seat is there because he will not fit into an economy seat, complain to the flight attendants that you will not be able to get past this hulk should it fall asleep, or in case of emergency. Inform them of your bladder condition. Insist that you be relocated or your seats be swapped. Aisle seats are preferable—unless you happen to be passing over Antarctica on a clear day.

If a neighbor can hear your headphones, you are playing them too loud.

If you can hear their headphones and they will not make the necessary adjustment, ask the flight attendant for another seat. Although the plane is likely to be full, you can usually get the flight attendants to side with you in a dispute with a rude neighbor. Simply report the infraction and, if necessary, inform the flight attendant what the offensive person said about their appearance, adding "I, myself, think you look very nice."

I have had good fortune in enlisting the aid of flight attendants. Once when a woman seated behind me was removing the nail polish from her lacquer-extruded claws with an open bottle of acetone—an instant migraine—I almost succeeded in having the offender and her petlike boyfriend arrested. They made the mistake of challenging the authority of the flight attendants whom I had enlisted through courtesy and admiring looks, not to mention reason, and had to be set straight by a copilot. In such close quarters even cloying perfume can be construed as an assault.

Conversations with seatmates should be confined to: "Excuse me," "Thank you," and "Pardon me." You have enough friends. There are exceptions, of course, as you may find yourself with an attractive, charming, and/or intelligent seatmate, but even then, conversation should be initiated with care. Remember, you can't get up and move should you get into a disagreement over Bush, Obama, or Brangelina. If your neighbor can't take a hint and persists in jabbering, smile and say nothing. Or feign narcoleptic sleep.

Turbulence

It is not OK to cry on the plane. Even if it's crashing and they're playing *Brian's Song*. In fact, it is imperative to keep a stiff upper lip when flying conditions are less than ideal, such as when severe turbulence is encountered or the plane is spiraling toward Earth. I have lived through numerous episodes of turbulence severe enough to cause luggage compartments to disgorge their contents, movie projectors to drop from the ceilings, and passengers to cry out or begin sobbing. During such times it is important not to join in the chorus of panicked shrieks, gasps, and ulu-lations emitted by the Nervous Nellies, but to see the turbulence in its proper perspective: fun. Haven't you ever been on the Cyclone at Coney Island?

I lost my fear of flying completely when I saw the sequence of Sam Shepard as Chuck Yeager test-piloting the X-1 in *The Right Stuff*. Just imagine that the horrific bouncing of your flight is due to its attempt to break the sound barrier, or think of it as an amusement park ride for which you paid ten bucks in northern Florida. Try to keep your eyes on the movie, and ask for a coaster to place over your drink so it won't spill. If necessary switch to white wine, Champagne, or vodka, which won't stain your clothing.

Borders

When you arrive in another country, you may not be welcomed with open arms, as Americans once tended to be, perhaps because of attitudinal retaliation over our country's tendency to humiliate the citizens of even our closest allies.

I suggest that whenever you arrive at the immigration desk that you remove your sunglasses, smile, and greet the agents politely in their own lan-guage. No matter what reason you may have for visiting the country, tell them you are a tourist. When asked for your occupation, always say "executive." Never list your profession as journalist, as you might as well write "spy."

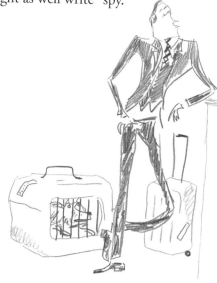

ON BLACK AND WHITE

I've been a puppet, a pauper, a pirate, a poet, a pawn, and a king. Occasionally, I've been the man. But I've never been a gangsta rapper and I'm OK with that.

I am not your average youth-culture cat, having been young so long it's old. I remember John Coltrane live at Slug's. I saw Hendrix and The Velvets live. I bought an advance ticket for Woodstock (dumb?). Yet I feel relatively unscathed by time. In 1991, while driving across America, I stopped in Albuquerque, New Mexico, and walked into a record store and hummed "Smells Like Teen Spirit" loudly until the clerk nodded and handed me the Nirvana CD.

I don't think I'm young, and I'm not faking it, but my senses still work well. You might see me at Other Music in the East Village buying Gnarls Barkley or the Boredoms, but mostly I listen to Bill Evans, Miles Davis, Thelonious Monk, Roland Kirk—music like that. My interest in hip-hop sort of petered out with Public Enemy, but if you see a Mercedes-Benz station wagon blasting "Fuck tha Police" or the bluegrass version of "Gin and Juice," that could be me.

I'm not really into youth, but I find myself allied with them out of mutual hatred of their parents. The enemy of my enemy is my friend. I bet Sonic Youth agrees, and they're about as wrinkled as I am.

This is all a sort of preamble. One day I was walking up Lafayette Street in Manhattan, and when I got to the Supreme shop I looked in the window as usual to see if anything caught my eye. (Hey, you don't have to be young to want a skateboard deck by John Baldessari.) Then I passed the other "street fashion" boutiques in the neighborhood, like Stackhouse and Brooklyn Industries, this being the board-culture B-boy fashion strip. I'm ambling and I hear a loud talker overtaking me. It was the kind of loud talk that signals a mobile phony, but this one was transmitting in rad Ebonics: "Yo, I be shoppin' fuh kicks, nigga, and all I be seein' is dis corny-ass designa shit… I ain't on 'at… I be headin' ova ta Modell's ta see if dey got some dope kicks…"

Theoretically, this hardened speech should have been emanating from a member of the 50 Cent entourage or at least a gun-toting gangsta outta Rikers, but yo, something was wrong, you know what I mean? There were too many NPM (niggaz-per-minute), and the sheer absence of adverbs, the lack of the subjunctive, the high quotient of simple progressive (he buyin'), the intensified continuatives (I be mad chillin'), the dropped copulas, and the multiple negations meant this language was too much. De-fuckin'-Trop, man! In other words, the cat be frontin' on an ill identity level.

I turned and, yes, it was a young white man dressed in shorts, sneakers, and a T-shirt. Kind of a plain look; no Ali G here. But that was the point of what he was broadcasting. He was not interested in street fashion because it was not "street" enough. I think he was suggesting that Supreme and 255 Studio (the limited-edition Nike shop) and Nom de Guerre and Stussy and Union were all fashion and no street. He wanted the dope projects shit.

"Street fashion" is big business, and youth have taken sneakers and T-shirts and turned them into a fashion codex as ruthlessly and absurdly driven by exclusivity and arbitrary, hollow one-upsmanship as the straight fashion world with its designer cults and conspicuous consumption signifiers. Every few months, I see a queue of young men, a few hundred maybe, camped out in front of Supreme ready to spend an entire night waiting for the new limited-edition kicks. It's a mixed bunch—blacks, whites, and a more-than-average proportion of Asians, especially Japanese. It seems that some of these guys are not themselves fashion desperadoes but entrepreneurs who can resell those limited-edition trainers on eBay to the real fashion desperadoes in Japan for several times what they paid.

Whither authenticity? I wondered with a melancholy air. I also wondered if this young Caucasian copycat would have continued in this verbal vein had I resembled Mike Tyson. How does this paleface, whose every other word was "nigger," respond to the presence of actual blacks? I would never know the answer to this, but I found such blatant wanksterism troubling.

I understand where this is coming from, aa-ight? White middle-class youth need someone to look up to, and sometimes maybe The White Stripes aren't enough. There is a craving for authenticity and realness and life-and-death struggles and they don't have any to call their own. The beatniks are gone. And the old hipsters on Schedule 1 narcotics are dead or on methadone maintenance. And the Weathermen blew themselves up. The punks are writing memoirs and doing oldies concerts. So what's a motherfucker to do?

In 1957, Norman Mailer published an essay entitled "The White Negro" in *Dissent* magazine. In it he wrote:

A totalitarian society makes enormous demands on the courage of men, and a partially totalitarian society makes even greater demands for the general anxiety is greater. Indeed if one is to be a man, almost any kind of unconventional action often takes disproportionate courage. So it is no accident that the source of Hip is the Negro, for he has been living on the margin between totalitarianism and democracy for two centuries.

Mailer saw the beat generation lift language from blacks via jazz. A later generation of hipsters reverently co-opted rhythm and blues and the blues. The Rolling Stones were a perfect manifestation of Mailer's White Negro, taking the music of Slim Harpo, Don Covay, and Chuck Berry and translating it through every fiber of their art-school Anglo-Saxon beings into something quite new and thrilling. Other musicians created similarly strange hybrids, such as Led Zeppelin with their Celtic Twilight–Howling

Wolf–Aleister Crowley fusion and The Yardbirds with their radioactive Sonny Boy Williamson. It was rock and roll and we liked it. It did everything culture is supposed to do—it gave us the tools to mutate with.

It wasn't a one-way street. Jazz itself was a fusion of European and African music. And in fact, jazz was a less satisfactory model for the emerging hipster, which Mailer saw as a new class of self-conscious psychopaths. Jazz was too sophisticated, too eloquent and articulate. What the rocker liked about blacks was what his parents feared about them. He liked their rejection of middle-class fashion in favor of stylized pimpwear (while the cool jazz men wore elegant suits). And then hip-hop presented an even more irresistible aspiration for bored white youth: the gangster, a violent antisocial without ideology acting entirely for his own immediate gratification. Hip-hop was armed and extremely dangerous, anti-idealistic, anti-intellectual, and anti-social. And so it was seen as bad (i.e., good).

Gangsta rap had a confluence of audiences attracted to the ultramasculine pose without content, which diverted attention from the progressive hip-hop of Public Enemy, De La Soul, the Jungle Brothers, Disposable Heroes, etc. But then funny things happened as characters like Jay-Z, Puffy Combs, and OutKast emerged, clouding the picture with their blatantly refined taste and flagrant upward mobility. P. Diddy be sittin' wit' Anna Wintour. What's a wigger to do?

Give up, dude. There is a place in hip-hop for Whitey, as the Beastie Boys proved with their twenty-four-track stand-up irony and as Eminem proved with his excoriating self-analysis and all-inclusive satire, but Whitey is never going to be a Crip or a Blood and instant gratification can't last. Marky Mark left the Funky Bunch behind and turned to keepin' it at least somewhat real. You've got to flow from within, like Bob Marley or Kurt Cobain or Lenny Bruce or Frank Sinatra—that's the only way to keep it real. That's life. Kick off those limited-edition kicks, put on some Lou Rawls, and feel the warmth of the melting pot, flowing toward a better future.

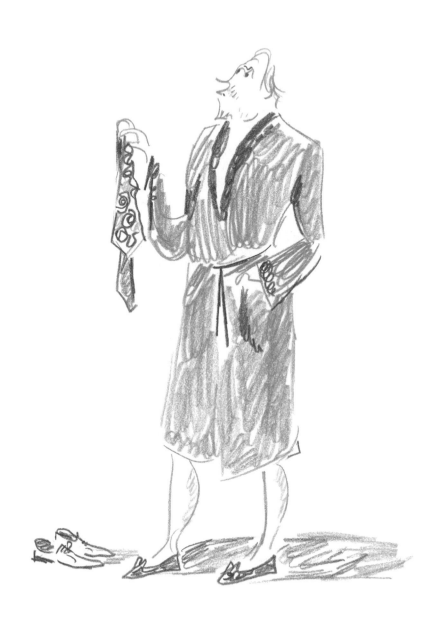

ON TASTE

"Taste is the fundamental quality which sums up all the other qualities. It is the ne plus ultra of the intelligence. Through this alone is genius the supreme health and balance of all the faculties."

—Comte de Lautréamont

To have taste. To have no taste. To be. Not to be. Taste is always the question and the answer, from the moment we awake until consciousness drops its trousers in the arms of Morpheus.

Taste is the most vital of our standards. We pride ourselves on our lack of prejudice, but who are we kidding? We may be color-blind, sexually ambivalent, culturally catholic, and tolerant of all forms of religious foolishness that don't infringe on our own aspirations to divinity, but when it comes to taste we are quite ruthless. Violate our personal canon of taste and our social defenses will rise and you will find yourself dropped like a hot potato. We are not here to determine your guilt or innocence, your worth or worthlessness, your intelligence or stupidity, but on the other hand we can't help but notice what you're wearing. Your taste is in our face.

Somehow taste sums up what a person is thinking and not thinking. Your carpet and drapes tell us more about you than anything you could possibly say. The books on your shelf, the black plastic twirling on your turntable, the condiment rack in your fridge, your sock drawer: these are the auguries by which we navigate society. Taste is the fingerprint of intelligence and the visible manifestation of personality. It's not a matter of reason or choice; taste attracts or repels us magnetically and automatically. If we ignore you, pardon our automatism. Our tastes come from the core of our beings, and when they change, I suspect the changes resonate in our very DNA. Taste is, in a way, our job on Earth. It's the machinery of human evolution. Bad taste leads to a biological cul de sac, extinction through shunning.

When we talk taste it is generally on the basis of observations made in the realm of eyeballing, not vintage sipping. It's the eye, not the tongue that is the principal organ of taste—but we can't forget where the idea of taste comes from. Taste comes from the mouth, not from just the taste buds that guard our pieholes but from the lips and tongue that execute our pronouncements of style.

Taste, the sense by which we discern food and beverage, has given its name to the overarching judgment of the senses acting in concert, which represents our personality. We say that someone has a good eye, but that doesn't quite capture the same range as good taste. We rarely say "He has a good ear" except in a musicological context, or "She has a great nose." Well, not usually anyway. And saying that someone has good touch usually implies skill in billiards or, say, surgery.

It's taste that says it all. The sense that is usually listed last of the five seems most akin to the sixth: ESP. Although it suggests the mouth, taste, in the sense of good or bad, is the product of all six portals to the outside world. Why? Is it the most complex? Certainly sight and sound present a variety and depth of display to the sensorium that is more complex than the gamut of flavor. Touch is arguably more pleasing, at least when the erotic is considered. It may be because taste, being intimately associated with sustenance, is seen as a matter of life and death. Taste protects us from poison and illness. And so when someone is judged as having bad taste there is something malicious about them. They are culturally toxic and generally we sense that they are to be avoided, unless we can change them—hopefully from a safe distance—if not remedying their affliction, at least shielding us from its perception.

There's something to the notion of healing bad taste in the practice of art and the creation of fashion. Mass taste is generally held in contempt or at least suspicion, but rather than fleeing it by any means necessary we tend to seek to alter it and elevate it, even if that is a hopeless task. Why do we persist in such foolish optimism? Maybe we fear that in democracies bad taste may be legislated.

Taste is a measure of culture. Taste started in the mouth, then took over the governance of the sensorium. Culture started on the farm and now it rules the metropolis, because culture was the perfect metaphor for how society grows, diversely and organically, even in its most artificial manifestations. Taste is our husbandry of culture. It's how we manage life itself on the most immediate and instinctive level. It is the early warning system of our reason.

We live in an empire of signs, demarcated in manners both explicit and inscrutable. And in the age of democracy, status and position are neither fixed nor as explicit as they were throughout human history. Hierarchies are often covert. Rank is negotiable. Taste, imperfectly perceived, is one of the chief systems of ranking.

Bad taste is universally derided, by most of its possessors and even by its flaunters. But good taste is a more sinister enemy. Good taste is established, safe, and static. "A man of great common sense and good taste, meaning thereby a man without originality or moral courage," wrote Mr. George Bernard Shaw. Voltaire decreed "The best is the enemy of the good." Rigid taste is the mark of rigid personality, a static position that breeds fatality. Decorator taste is personality by proxy. If it's not a lie, it's capitulation.

Taste should always be slightly disturbing or unsettling. There is a shock that comes from the authentically new. I remember hearing a Rolling

Stones single for the first time and reacting negatively, not understanding it. My ears were offended. Two or three listens later I was awed. The most interesting taste presents itself as a problem to be solved, and it makes one think. The best taste, as opposed to good taste, is imperfect, unfinished, experimental, a work in progress. Taste proceeds from instinct adjusted by the scientific method: trial and error. Great taste is brave taste, frightening housewives and coddled children. Great taste leads by amazing, astounding, and perplexing. It adjusts the zeitgeist. It takes a little time to take effect, and when the perceiver understands the possessor may have already moved on. As William Wordsworth said of his friend Samuel Coleridge: "Every great and original writer, in proportion as he is great and original, must himself create the taste by which he is to be relished." The same, of course, can be said for every great and original artist, musician, and dandy.

Popular taste is a problem, whether it is considered bad or good. Bad taste is often preferable to good taste because it may possess certain virtues, such as daring and exuberance. Good taste tends toward fascism and monotony, and its mechanisms are often bullying and destructive. Those of self-proclaimed good taste see it as their duty to keep out the low and vulgar elements, to guard the gates of the club and to ensure that certain potentially stimulating and edifying activities take place only behind closed doors. Such fancy taste is a strange hybrid of morality and publicity. But even when taste presents itself as a positive value, it may be extraordinarily flawed.

In *The Theory of the Leisure Class,* Thorstein Veblen posited the principles of conspicuous consumption and conspicuous waste as the key mechanisms of status in the modern class system. It has been more than a hundred years since Veblen wrote:

The requirement of conspicuous wastefulness is not commonly present, consciously, in our canons of taste, but it is none the less present as a constraining norm, selectively shaping and sustaining our sense of what is beautiful,

and guiding our discrimination with respect to what may legitimately be
approved as beautiful and what may not.

What would Veblen think of the ten-thousand-square-foot McMansions and behemoth paramilitary vehicles of the lower-upper class? What
would he think of braggarts posing as poets, armed with automatic
weapons and decked out in hideous gewgaws encrusted in South African
diamonds? I suppose he would be an instant convert to the theory of
de-evolution. We seem to have reached the epitome of waste culture,
and even when we are clearly threatened with a fatal revolt of nature, we
insist on the display of waste as a cultural signifier. Egad!

Obviously we need a taste revolution. What it will look like is complicated. It will not be Casual Friday, that fake leveling trend that is really a way
to camouflage and codify wealth and power—taking us from conspicuous
consumption to cryptic consumption. Taste must be green. And it must be
modest, in the root sense. Taste is about proper measure. And undoubtedly
taste must turn away from the luxury trademarks of conglomerates gone wild
toward a cultivated, proportionate, personal sensibility where the artisanship
of cottage industry replaces the brute force of the mechanical production line.

The designer and programmer Paul Graham wrote an interesting
essay called "Taste for Makers" in 2002, in which he made the case for an
objective, almost scientific sense of beauty to inform design. He noted that
Copernicus's initial objections to Ptolemy's cosmology were aesthetic.
And he quoted Ben Rich, designer of the Stealth aircraft:

All of us had been trained by Kelly Johnson [designer of the P-38, F-80,
F-104 and U-2] and believed fanatically in his insistence that an airplane that
looked beautiful would fly the same way.

In recent years modernism in design has returned, good old-
fashioned modernism, not the chaotic postmodern stunts of Frank Gehry

or the hogwild phallic totemism of Cesar Pelli, but the measured, optimistic futurism of Neutra, Eames, and Saarinen. There's no reason why something can't look new world but still express Vitruvius's principles of symmetry. And suddenly the reverence for nature shown by Frank Lloyd Wright and Russel Wright seems relevant again with a new generation of green architects. Taste is a survival instinct. Not everyone will survive.

Taste is especially crucial today, because consumer society defines personality less through behavior, expression, and the creative process than through the unnatural selection of brand-name fashion fealty. Although real personality is more than a container full of logos, it is still considered important to fly the right colors in the dangerously shallow waters of fashion.

Emperors, except the current nude ones, have always had their tasters. And still they have managed to get poisoned. There are no trustworthy taste accountants. The decorator works for himself first. Taste must be personal, intimate, and alive, responding in a moment. In today's world we can't trust the pro tasters—they've been bought off. We have to be our own tasters, finding our own beautiful, exquisite, harmonious, and witty way through the wastelands of the unpalatable. We don't necessarily want our taste to be tasteful, but we can't help smiling when somebody says, "That's tasty!"

HOW TO BE FAMOUS (OR NOT)

"A celebrity is one who is known by many people he is glad he doesn't know."

—H. L. Mencken

"I handle fame by not being famous. I'm not famous to me."

—Bob Marley

For thousands upon thousands of years, we lived under caste and class systems that segmented society hierarchically. Slobs down there, swells up here. One was either noble or common, and never the twain met, at least in broad daylight. But then invention and exploration led to a mercantile society and commoners began to accumulate wealth. Then the social revolutions of the nineteenth century led to a republican democracy, which more or less eliminated the aristocrats, as we had known them throughout history. Royals and nobles would still exist, as a sort of quaint tourist attraction, but new upper classes arose, defined by the yardsticks of achievement. The right to rule was no longer God-given; it was won by fame.

Today we live in what is regarded as a democracy. The people, or the majority of them, are theoretically endowed with wisdom, and they rule through elected representatives. If mankind is good and not evil, then fifty-one percent of men must be right, or so the theory goes. In ancient Athens and Rome, democracy never quite functioned up to the ideals of theory, and there was a tendency toward demagoguery, scandal, and war. Sometimes bad things happened to good people, as in the case of Socrates, yet democracy, a system designed to function at the level of villages, persists today as the accepted ideal government of enormous states.

In early democracy, political units were small and the citizens knew one another. Aristotle said:

"If the citizens of a state are to judge and distribute offices according to merit, then they must know each others' characters; where they do not possess this knowledge, both the election to offices and the decision of lawsuits will go wrong."

In vast, modern democracies it is impossible for the citizens to know much about one another, and yet we persist in believing that the majority will make wise choices.

Why? Well, to not believe it would be…undemocratic. So the basic premise of our system is never questioned because the alternative would be to admit that aristocracy or oligarchy had its advantages. Walter Lippmann wrote:

In this deadly conflict between their ideals and their science, the only way out was to assume without much discussion that the voice of the people was the voice of God.[1]

The hope of resolving this problem of democracy was in the perfection of a mass media, which would enable the citizens to know one another better, making the state a smaller, more well-informed place. It would also create the possibility of mass manipulation of the people through the new science of public relations, but hopefully the voice of God would win out over the propaganda machines.

Today we seem to be heading toward a new kind of state, where a celebrity class functions as a new form of nobility. Not that there will ever be a television show called *I'm a Viscount, Get Me Out of Here* or *Nobility Apprentice*, but celebrity is functional aristocracy, a new elect. The House of Celebrities hasn't yet replaced the House of Lords, but stranger things have happened. You can go from playing Conan the Barbarian one day to Governor of California the next. Fame is like money—it is liquid currency and it can be put to many uses. And where fame was once sought only by a few, it is now the obsession of the masses, millions of them hoping to be famous for at least a quarter of an hour.

Children who once grew up wanting to be a doctor, a lawyer, or a soldier now grow up with a single ambition: to be famous. By any means necessary. Everybody wants it. It's the ticket out of Nowheresville. One day you're hosting a Western on TV shilling 20 Mule Team Borax, and the next day you're in the Oval Office. It's a miracle. It must be that that same God who speaks infallibly through the people has touched you, transforming you into a celebrity, a being who lives in another sphere. It's secular sainthood by acclamation. But fame can come with a terrible price. Privacy does not exist for the public figure. Your life belongs to the masses and your fame can easily turn to notoriety, to infamy.

The best fame is probably the kind that pays well without making one universally recognized, meaning that one can lead a normal life, transiting public spaces without harassment. It is better to be Dan Brown than Tony Soprano. Most of the typical forms of insanity that afflict celebrities derive from their constantly being recognized and accosted by strangers. Suddenly this fact of life affects much of their waking time, making them feel targeted and vulnerable. If fear is real, it's not paranoia.

This said, many celebrities imagine their effect on the public to be greater than it is. I have walked with numerous undisguised famous persons and I have found that the best defense against being recognized is being unexpected. I remember walking two dozen blocks on the West Side with Madonna Ciccone and she wasn't recognized once. She was wearing a baseball cap, but I believe if you turn off your aura you can go anywhere without being noticed (except the subway).

The most problematic aspect of being famous is that it engenders a significant cult of people who would see you utterly destroyed, if not physically then in your reputation and career. The press builds you up to tear you down, just because they feel they have to and they can. Others are simply jealous: what have you got that they don't? If you are destroyed, that means your slot is vacant. Despite the downside, and the ignominy that haunts the ex-celebrity, everyone still wants to be famous. They'll do anything to get there. Anything.

But think about it. Do you want to be followed by paparazzi? Paparazzi in recklessly driven autos stalking you to your favorite bistro? Do you want a helicopter hovering over your wedding? Do you want your significant other and you referred to with a combination name by the tabloids (as in Bennifer, Brangelina, Tomkat)? Do you want groupies hiding in your shrubbery, suddenly bursting out of a bush, their cameras strobing stars onto your retinas and testing the resilience of your coronary arteries?

Is the notoriety worth it? Really?

Do you want to worry about your wineglass being stolen so fans can clone you from your DNA? Do you want your wineglass photographed after you get out of rehab? Do you want every ugly detail of your horrendous divorce recounted in the tabloids and commented on by Cindy Adams and Andrea Peyser? Do you want every unintentional kiss of the wrong person or slip on a banana peel or a medication reported in Page Six, or worse—if there is worse?

Are you sure?

Do you want your sexual preferences questioned on *South Park*? Do you want that casual one-night stand to result in conception? Do you want pictures in the paper of you screaming at your kids? Do you want the price of everything jacked up? Do you want everyone in every restaurant staring at you and the spinach stuck in your teeth? Do you want to be followed into the bathroom by autograph seekers? Do you want that ten percent tip in the newspaper? Do you want to be a plus fifteen instead of plus one? I thought not.

Fame may make a few things better. But it makes most things far, far worse. Like your chances of being approved by the co-op board, getting those expensive or illicit items through customs, getting a real stock tip, having dinner with a person who is not actually your spouse, getting your kids into particularly discreet schools or yourself into a low-key country club, being discovered using controversial prescriptions or even the ones everyone else takes, like Viagra or Valium, or making a slip of the pencil on your income tax. Death. Any rudeness or unkindness is magnified tenfold. Every subpar gratuity or grumpy retort is national news. Lies told about you will tend to be given credence simply because it makes good news copy. But above all, most people who read about you will be jealous of your beauty, your talent, and your good fortune; and they will all be rooting for your utter ruin: your impoverishment, your physical debilitation, your arrest, trial, and incarceration, and most likely, your painful, ignominious death and your utter oblivion to future generations.

I know it would be easy to give in and become a household name, but don't do it. Find a nice comfy niche in the lower ranks of notoriety and stay there. I have.

When it comes to avoiding fame, rule number one is: avoid having your name in the paper. At the dawning of the age of publicity, it was said that ladies and gentlemen had their names in the newspaper three times: once when they were born, once when they were married, and once when they died. Of course in the information age this is impractical, and one should make allowances for at least two or three marriages and the appropriate number of divorces. And we can make allowances for one or two indictments.

How do you avoid the newspaper? Never respond to requests for quotations or comments even though you are eminently qualified to do so and have something intelligent to say while others around you are blithering. "No comment!" is pretentious and, worse, likely to be noted. "Who does he think he is, not commenting!" Simply become incoherent: "Well, I suppose that given the circumstances...I mean...any way you look at it...there are bound to be...well... that all depends...who can say, really?"

The best defense against fame is to act as a famous person never would. Insanity is no safety net; celebrities often behave irrationally.

Humility will throw celebrity chasers off the scent every time. And intellectual behavior is a sure sign that you are nobody. Quote Chomsky, Lacan, Baudrillard, and, if you're desperate, Henry James.

If you do get approached by paparazzi, no need to hold a newspaper over your face, as in a perp-walk situation; simply close your eyes. They'll never use the blink shot. If you are going to be riding in a car, always wear underwear. Always give the wrong name to the photographer who took your picture, and make it a generic name, like John Smith or Juan Sanchez Jr. Many things may be written about you, but due to certain loopholes in the system, most publications still insist on publishing facts, and so when the fact-checkers call, remember: deny everything. Fact-checkers are usually young people, little skilled in deception, and they take no greater pleasure than deleting passages from a writer's account of things. Remember: you didn't say it, that was somebody else, and you were somewhere else entirely at the time; you never heard of the person quoting you, and, in fact, you are one of identical triplets.

Certain professions should be studiously avoided: big-time crime or criminal law, politics, usury, slumlording. Show-business careers are not necessarily out of the question, but acting and the hip-hop industry are inadvisable choices. Mime, string quartets, Shakespeare, and all forms of dance except lap are fairly safe. Avoid professions where a vow of chastity and/or poverty is required unless you can keep it. Academia is fairly risk free. Becoming a poet, novelist, or jazz musician almost ensures a high degree of anonymity. No one will ever know who you are. Safe hobbies to pursue: philosophy, philately, bird-watching, numismatics, and sports like curling or croquet.

But if you have achieved something of note or significance, simply credit others. People will think that you are insane and therefore uninteresting, which is a condition of complete safety.

In most cases, thinking stealthily is the key. Look at our military's bombers. They are stealth bombers. Their edge is not speed or power but going undetected. Do they want to be famous? Certainly not. Anonymity is a strategy. Develop a set of nicknames for yourself and your friends. Talk in code like the fellows in that imaginary group the Cosa Nostra. Use dated slang, like that of early-twentieth-century jazzmen or pimps. Never say anything that can be understood by an eavesdropper. Do not attend reunions or join alumni associations. If your spouse is threatening to become famous, adopt another name or change the spelling of yours.

The key to freedom is being invisible. William S. Burroughs, who managed to be famous while being generally unrecognized, said the key to invisibility is seeing the other person first. Burroughs became famous in his old age, whereupon he moved to Kansas to preserve his anonymity, as those who knew him were likely to be found on either coast. Johnny Carson always vacationed in Europe, where he was virtually unknown.

Should you happen to be a real estate developer, do not put your name on your buildings. Even if you are not a real estate developer, do not own a modeling agency, or put out a bottled water or vodka with your name and face on it.

If you become a blogger or participate in Internet chat, don't use your real name. Do not attempt to meet people on the Internet, even if they claim to be over eighteen. If you must be on a social network, do it under an assumed name and keep your content fictional.

The truth is for your friends, and sometimes it's hard to tell who they are. If you become famous, the incentives to betray you are multiplied exponentially. Information should be given out on a need-to-know basis; tell them what you need them to know, but if you tell more than one person, alter the version slightly so that when it is made public you'll know the identity of the culprit. Whenever possible, downplay your interesting and glamorous qualities. I remember going to a party with Jean-Michel Basquiat shortly before he became unavoidably famous. When approached by people intrigued by his appearance and asked what he did for a living, he would reply, "I'm the manager of a McDonald's." A perfect conversation stopper.

Discretion is said to be the better part of valor. The better part of discretion is candor and/or modesty, the sure sign of a regular person and a noncelebrity. To avoid fame, always attempt to tell the truth unless it's nobody's business, exhibit impeccable manners, and care about those less fortunate. Relevance is your ticket out of the limelight. "Why is irrelevancy so often taken for profundity?" asked Fairfield Porter. Avoid irrelevancy at all costs. Ask tough questions. Be sincere and earnest. Know the facts. You will usually scare off those who would put you in jeopardy through their gratuitous glorification of you.

If you feel the temptation to do something idealistic or charitable, for God's sake keep it under your hat. Make anonymous donations and avoid charity balls and benefit auctions.

Many celebrities talk about keeping it real. This is a tip-off that you should never keep it blatantly real. As Les McCann sang, "Trying to make it real compared to what?" Always leave them guessing. Bono may be real and relevant, and he's famous for that. It's unlikely anyone else can get away with it. Refer them to Bono. He's got good security. If you must be an upright, honorable, and idealistic person, don't let on.

But don't take my word for it. I could be lying.

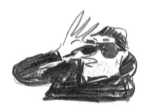

1   *Public Opinion*, Walter Lippman, 1922.

HOW TO DEAL WITH DIVINITY (OR NOT)

"The most common of all follies is to believe passionately in the palpably not true. It is the chief occupation of mankind."

—H. L. Mencken

"Science is the record of dead religions."

—Oscar Wilde

If you are a religious person, you may wish to move on to the next chapter. Or book. If you are a religious person, you probably have your mind made up and anything I have to say on the subject is unlikely to interest you. This chapter is intended primarily for those who are surrounded by religious persons but are not themselves religious.

Politics and religion are two things often best avoided as topics of conversation. Why? For one thing, you can't win. Also conversations aren't usually held with the object of coming to the truth but to pass the time, and time is best passed pleasantly. Religion is a subject that people kill one other over.

In some parts of the world, religion is clearly losing its power. In France, a third of the population believes in neither a God nor a spirit or life force. In Germany, a quarter of the population is atheist, in Britain one in five people are. But in Turkey only one in one hundred would call himself an atheist, and in other Muslim countries, no one would dare. There are nine countries where Sharia, or Islamic law based on the Koran, is the law of the land. In the United States, the state of belief is closer to Turkey's than Western Europe's. Americans are religious and tend to be intolerant of those who are not. Polls show that a majority of Americans would not vote for an atheist—apparently it's worse than being gay for a politician. Yet over the last half century church attendance has fallen off sharply and scandal has plagued the mighty Roman Catholic Church. Things are changing.

With the threat of global communism vanished, the tensions in the world today can be mainly ascribed to religious conflict. Even for those personally unconcerned with religion, it is the nine-hundred-pound gorilla in the room (wearing a turban, mitre, or yarmulke). Religion is aggressive. It may be receding in many cities and suburbs, but elsewhere it is growing, militantly proselytizing and waging wars of expansion. Even in America someone may knock on your door in the hope of enlisting you in their faith.

When one is unwillingly subjected to proselytizing, it is best to nip things in the bud in as simple a manner as possible. If Jehovah's Witnesses or Mormons come knocking on your door, then treat them as you would any other unsolicited solicitor. Turn them away.

But religion is hard to escape. Even if you are a known atheist, you will find yourself attending events of a religious nature or aspect, such as marriages, christenings, bar and bas mitvahs, and funerals. You may even find yourself invited to a seder. I always enjoy a seder because I like the food, the singing, and any meal that requires you to drink four glasses of wine. And I don't mind the ritual any more than I mind when my kid has *SpongeBob Squarepants* on the television. The best approach to social religion is to play along. Humor them. Enjoy!

But if you're known as a doubter or unbeliever, it's best not to push it. I think I went too far not long ago when, after a few drinks, I took Communion at a Catholic wedding. Several persons in the party knew that I had not attended an entire Mass since 1966, and they might have been surprised that I did not burst into flames. No more Communion for me.

My philosophy is to go to the church or temple, dress properly, wear the yarmulke, sit when they sit, stand when they stand. I don't kneel. Only American Catholics kneel. It's not just my sports-eroded knees; I find it a little on the dramatic, "hair shirt" side of religious practice.

And don't ask me to pray. I kind of go along with the old Jim Morrison line: "You cannot petition the Lord with prayer." I mean you can, sure, but you can also talk to yourself with much the same effect. William Blake wrote: "Prayer is the study of art." That I can go along with.

It's funny, because I do like ritual. I like a well-acted and well-sung High Mass. And I confess I've got a soft spot for polytheism, particularly in its Greek and Roman forms. I prefer the classical stories to those of the Judeo-Christian book. The gods, God bless 'em, are not always right. They get horny. They get angry. They fuck up. They're just like us except they live forever.

For some reason, these ancient gods are considered much more unbelievable than the One God Who is Three Persons, one of whom was born to a virgin. But I say it all depends on what you can believe in. Personally I find the exploits of Zeus, Athena, Apollo, Hermes, Aphrodite, and the rest of the Olympian gang as believable as those of God the Father and His Son. And the old pantheon certainly seems at least as believable the current incumbents. The Greek gods became unpopular for one reason or another and lost out to a competition smart enough to appropriate the old gods as saints. Gods, uppercase or lowercase, are like Tinkerbell, the fairy in *Peter Pan*. She was able to live because she was believed in. I think that if we began to believe in the Olympian pantheon again, the gods would be delighted to return and continue their adventures, taking lust, anger, vengeance, and treachery to new, postmodern heights.

Having been raised in "the one true faith" and subsequently entered with enthusiasm the real world, I have a skeptical view of religion. I don't like one true faiths or chosen people—or master races, for that matter. I believe in the melting pot, and that goes for deities too. The Romans had the right idea. If a hot, new god came along from some far-flung part of the empire, they just added him or her to the list. Isis? Why not? Mithra? I know the perfect spot for his temple. If divinity exists outside of the human imagination, then there is far too much divine work to be done for there to be only one god. If I'm going to go along with one god, I'm going to go along with them all, sort of the way the Haitians do it.

Forced to choose a faith, I would have to select Olympian, although I have never seen that as a box to check off on an application or form. I guess Olympians are supposed to answer to "pagan," but that's a kind of derisive term, being derived from the Latin *paganus*, meaning "rustic" or "hick." And if you call yourself a pagan, people might think you are a Wiccan, which I find a little Halloweeny for my taste. Today the ancient Greeks' and Romans' beliefs are misunderstood and portrayed as superstition. It is clear from the writings of those such as Cicero that sophisticated polytheists also had an uppercase "G" god, but that their prime mover, like that of Enlightenment deists, was considered to be so abstract and distant as to be irrelevant to day-to-day life.

Belief in the one, big, all-powerful uppercase God doesn't mean that we have to discard all the lowercase specialist gods, any more than believing in Jesus means you can't believe in Santa Claus. It's like saying we have a primary care physician, but then there are times when we need the dermatologist, the urologist, the ophthalmologist, and the ear, nose, and throat guy. The old gods were specialists.

Unfortunately, many of the leading religions, such as Judaism, Christianity, and Islam, insist that we have no other gods before us. A real spoilsport attitude, I think. I suppose this is good business practice for them, wiping out the competitors, but there's no reason that we should, in the twenty-first century, kowtow to second-millennium monopolists practicing monotheism. There is some truth to the label Islamofascism, just as there has been Christofascism and Judeofascism. It is the monolithic, monotheistic religions, the cartels of belief, that tend to behave violently toward those who do not share their beliefs.

And if people need religions, why should they have to be ancient? I admit that I consider most of the newer cults to be in rather bad taste, but they do have their points. Even the Scientologists have some good ideas; they just have a scary management style. Scientology is not considered a religion in Germany, France, Belgium, Canada, and the U.K. But who gets to say what a religion is? The Constitution of the United States says "Congress shall make no law respecting an establishment of religion," but then the IRS seems to feel entitled to grant tax-exempt status to this church, but not that church.

This seems totally at odds with "Novus ordo seclorum," the slogan on the great seal of our country. If this is a "new order for the ages," then isn't a new order of religion in order? Look at the new infrastructure of the world. Global instant communication has created a kind of giant hive brain that could be another kind of god if it managed to actually wake up. What if we are all cells in some giant intelligence that is just now being assembled through the medium of the electron? That's an idea that goes back to Nathaniel Hawthorne's 1851 novel *The House of the Seven Gables*: "Is it a fact—or have I dreamt it—that, by means of electricity, the world of matter has become a great nerve, vibrating thousands of miles in a breathless point of time? Rather, the round globe is a vast head, a brain, instinct with intelligence!"

H. G. Wells took up this idea and ran with it pretty far in his 1938 book *World Brain*, which envisioned a world encyclopedia (not dissimilar to Wikipedia meets Google). In fact the concept of the Internet is inherent in this book. These concepts were further fleshed out in Arthur C. Clarke's 1962 volume *Profiles of the Future*, in which he saw supercomputers as a practical organizing principle for Wells's "world brain," and in Douglas Hofstadter's 1979 book *Gödel, Escher, Bach*, which studies structures of intelligence and compares the brain to the collective intelligence of an ant colony.

Now that we have people orbiting up there "in Heaven" and we get to see our planet as a rotating unit, we may learn to profit from a different perspective. I agree with William S. Burroughs: "Anyone who prays in space is not *there*."[1]

In a democracy, the majority rules. In our democracy, the majority puts faith before the facts. And so despite what we know, we are still subject to ancient fictions that may prove powerful enough to trump the truth. If I have any faith, I place it in intelligence and beauty.

As for religion, I'll go along with a few answers provided by Ezra Pound in "Religio:"

> What is a god?
> A god is an eternal state of mind…
> When is god manifest?
> When the states of mind take form.
> When does a man become a god?
> When he enters one of these states of mind…
> By what characteristic may we know the divine forms?
> By beauty.[2]

1   William S. Burroughs, "It Is Necessary to Travel," in *The Adding Machine: Selected Essays* (New York: Seaver Books, 1986).

2   Ezra Pound, "Religio, or, The Child's Guide to Knowledge," in *Ezra Pound: Selected Prose 1909–1965* (New York: New Directions Publishing Corporation, 1973).

ON PATRIOTISM

We often hear about patriotism but we never hear about matriotism. Which is odd because there as many people who think of their nation as their mother country as those who regard their native turf as the fatherland. Actually, today the fatherland is out. It's too Nazi Germany. And mothering is in again, after decades of feminism and a rising Gaia consciousness. The Earth is alive! Yes, she is! There are a lot of earth mothers out there, and maybe they're poised to take over the planet.

Perhaps it's time for a change. After about four thousand years of male domination, maybe goddesses and queens are making a comeback. There are signs. Most of the countries where the term "fatherland" has been used now have female heads of state, such as Germany, Denmark, the Netherlands, and Iceland. There are heads of state who are women even in countries with a significant male majority, such as Bangladesh and India, the latter having 40 million more men in its population than women—a difference that is nearly equivalent to the entire population of Argentina.

Traditionally the earth is mother. The sky is father. Agriculture was a feminine occupation; hunting and war were male gigs. Nations took on a masculine personality because they liked to fight for more turf. So nations were always looking for a few good men, as in patriot heroes willing to make the ultimate sacrifice for their country: their lives. But times have changed. War has become too nasty a proposition, and it seems increasingly sensible and profitable to see one's country as something to develop and cultivate as a tourist destination instead of something to die for. But old habits die hard, and the idea of nationalism that was born in the eighteenth century is still with us, especially in countries like ours that believe they are not only the best in the world but have a destiny to lead the world. Or countries that believe they are on God's side, like the Islamic republics. Sometimes a nation believes they are a chosen people, an important tenet of Judaism that, under Christianity, was superlatively grafted on to Roman Catholicism, and to British imperial culture during the Romantic Age, when Britain saw itself as "the New Jerusalem." Just when things seem to be getting sophisticated around here, somebody starts seeing a city on a hill or a thousand points of light—and *boom!* Here we go again! It would be easy to regard the twentieth-century expressions of nationalism as old-fashioned and chauvinistic, except for the inconvenient jihad that casts America as the great Satan. War? What is it good for? Absolutely nothing. But we're stuck with it.

The upper classes, following in the footsteps of aristocracy, see themselves as citizens of the world. Patriotism is something to stir up among the help when it's good for business. It's really a quaint form of group self-aggrandization that appeals to the unsophisticated. But what's a motherland to do?

In the United States we have neither a fatherland nor a motherland but a homeland, at least ever since the United States Department of Homeland Security was established in 2002. "Homeland" struck me as a bizarre choice, sounding faintly...Rhodesian. I guess it was considered a nonsexist usage, but it made me feel like I was going to end up sent somewhere. I don't like the implications of "Security" in that title either. It makes me feel insecure. It would have been better if we had changed the Department of Defense back to the original, more accurate Department of War and called this new agency the Department of Defense, or perhaps Department of Defensiveness.

Americans have always been a patriotic lot. It took team spirit to drive out the French, to throw off the British crown, and to conquer and decimate an indigenous population now estimated as having originally been 50 to 100 million after centuries of euphemistic lowballing the estimate to justify filling up all that unused space. But of course history is written by the victors, and if you can say anything about Americans it is that they have been chronic victors, up until the Vietnam War anyway.

In the United States nationalism declined during the sixties as the hippie and antiwar movements spurred a new internationalism among the youth. But Old Glory and the national anthem still sanctified every sports event while the United States quietly finished taking over the white man's burden from Europe. Then, beginning with the dramatic Reagan administration and especially following the September 11 attacks, there was a rise of American exceptionalism, the theory that the United States plays a special role in history, having a unique destiny to lead the world to equality and democracy.

Ronald Reagan repeatedly paraphrased Jesus's Sermon on the Mount, characterizing America as "a shining city upon a hill." George H. W. Bush envisioned the magic republic with the metaphor of a thousand points of light, perhaps conjuring up the sublime view from space enjoyed by ICBMs. Americans are nation fetishists and have been ever since the days of Manifest Destiny. It doesn't say "Novus ordo seclorum" on the dollar bill for nothing. This was an egoist country from the beginning, self-consciously founded on the deist principles of the Enlightenment. Untouched by "divine right," the stage in America was clear for plutocracy.

Americanism, like some other forms of nationalism, took on religious overtones, which culminated with George W. Bush's unfortunate representation of "the war on terror" as a crusade on September 16, 2001. But the events of a few days earlier were sufficient enough to kick up American nationalism to old-fashioned wartime levels. However, with the world wired for audio and video there is ultimately no going back to old-school nationalism. With the threat of the Soviet Union gone, Europe unified, and China converted to big business, it's clear that internationalism is on the rise. Asked if he believed in American exceptionalism, Barack Obama replied, "I believe in American exceptionalism, just as I suspect that the Brits believe in British exceptionalism, and the Greeks believe in Greek exceptionalism."

But non-jingoists still have to tread softly. People have the big fear and they want to be safe from jihad by any means necessary. So wearing American flag lapel pins has gotten to be a big deal. Politicians don't leave home without them. In 2008, a reporter noticed that Barack Obama wasn't wearing one and Obama boldly explained that he had stopped wearing an American flag pin because he felt it had become "a substitute for, I think, true patriotism, which is speaking out on issues that are of importance to our national security. I decided I won't wear that pin on my chest." Then after months of hammering from right-wing pundits Obama began trotting the pin out occasionally.

I don't wear an American flag pin, and I don't have any magnetic ribbons on the back of my car. I don't fly an American flag at home because my home is not a fortress and it's in uncontested New England territory that is clearly in the domain of the United States of America. I believe that my actions, such as paying my taxes and rooting for the Yankees (not to mention the J-E-T-S, Jets, Jets, Jets!) demonstrate adequately that I am an American. My not wearing a flag on my lapel doesn't mean I'm an agent of international communism, but that I think allegiance is complicated.

When my ancestors were running short on potatoes, this country took them in. (Well actually, when my ancestors got bored with the cold in Canada, this country took them in.) And this country has been good to my family, going back to the early seventeenth century when my DNA first arrived on these shores. But let's not be rash. I am quite fond of the old sod of Eire as well. If I were to have a second passport, it would be that of the motherland of many of my ancestors. (Unfortunately all of my grandparents were born on this side of the pond, so until further genealogical research proves otherwise, I am without E.U. papers.)

I am an American patriot/matriot with a great tenderness for all of the sources of my genetic composition (which I have recently learned, thanks in part to the heroic genealogical efforts performed by the Church of Jesus Christ of Latter-day Saints in order to baptize by proxy the deceased):

Ireland, England, France, Germany, Alsace-Lorraine, the Holy Roman Empire, and the Roman Empire. (Not only am I descended, in all likelihood, from Brian Boru and Niall of the Nine Hostages, but I am also a descendant of Charlemagne and a couple of Roman emperors.) I am not above accumulating passports. No descendent of William the Conqueror and Charles Martel should have only one passport. I don't expect that we'll ever have to flee America, as Jews once had to flee Germany, but as we used to say in the Boy Scouts of America: "Be prepared." At the moment the leading contender for the 2012 Republican Presidential candidacy is not a rational person. And, truth be told, I do feel far more at home in Paris and Sicily than I do in about forty-four of our American states.

Politics is fantastic sport, but I have no interest in being more involved in it than voting. I vote on the premise that someday I may cast a deciding ballot, just as someday I may win the Mega Millions Lotto game. I prefer to think of politics as a gestalt or holistic thing, and my best political actions are things that most people would not regard as political at all. The way Beau Brummell dressed was political. Jasper Johns's American flag is political, as was Jimi Hendrix's arrangement of the "The Star-Spangled Banner." I think my blue shoes are political.

I want to make things work as much as the next guy, but I'm a citizen of the planet first and that's a position I recommend to all earthlings. And after that I probably consider myself a New Yorker and a New Englander. I'm not much of a New York State enthusiast because of the clowns in the state government in Albany, but I do like the new retro orange and blue license plates. And then, down the line, I am a patriotic citizen of the good old U.S.A. But I have my reservations.

I'm sorry, but I firmly believe in the scale effect, and it's quite possible that the United States of America as it is presently constituted is simply too large to govern elegantly. We've reached a state of uncritical mass. The Greeks invented democracy as a form of government for a political unit in which everyone knew everybody else. What we actually have is a media-ocracy, or mediocracy. We're ruled by televised fictions, and they're just not believable anymore.

The Soviet Union had the right idea when it devolved, making its constituent states sovereign. I advocate a sort of Hong Kong status for New York, and I believe the original thirteen colonies (with the possible addition of Florida and Louisiana) would make a nice, medium-size country to which I could easily pledge my allegiance. California and those two other wine-producing states on the Pacific would also make a great new nation. Texas has been threatening to become a nation practically from its beginning. And that great middle ground, well, wouldn't they be happier without our smug East Coast attitudes?

I'm just asking. As a patriot. And a matriot.

HOW TO AGE

"Getting old isn't so bad; it's nonexistence that hurts."

—Frank O'Hara

We live in a world of inverted values. Youth today is accorded the respect and admiration once given to age, and elders are despised or dismissed as irrelevant. Old is not in keeping with fashion or modernism in that old is not new and hence automatically better than anything we have ever seen before. So aging adults everywhere, feeling miserably past it, desperately resort to undignified strategies of liveliness in hope of being perceived as younger than they are.

Oh, the legions of mutton dressed as lamb! Oh, the hogs acting the piglet! Oh, the old goats cavorting as kids! Women can afford to have their faces painstakingly rebuilt to resemble those of their youth while men are exhorted to dye their hair and beards by former athletes and nagged to take pills that might produce erections lasting up to six hours.

Whereas once youths did all they could do to appear older and more mature, taking joy in putting on the long pants of manhood and treasuring those first few wisps of beard, mature adults today shave their pubic hair in imitation of pre-nubiles and costume themselves in the clothing of adolescent rebels. Yikes, Grandma is in go-go boots! What happened? How did the social order get turned so upside down?

It seems to have something to do with so-called youth culture. But youth *culture* doesn't exist. A youth *cult* certainly exists, and a youth *market* exists big-time, encompassing not only the young but also those who would be young—again and forever.

The idealization and idolization of youth pits the young and old against one another in a parody of class struggle. Fashion and art glorify youth for its own sake and lay the evils of the world at the feet of older generations. This serves only to distract us from the real villains. Youth is innocent? Age is guilty? Not! This corny mentality hit its stride with my generation, the baby boomers that became hippies and rebelled against the Vietnam War and placed their faith in sex, drugs, and rock and roll. We were told, "Don't trust anyone over thirty." They should have told us instead, "Don't trust anyone with over 30 million."

Youth culture (sic) generally advances the theme: I hope I die before I get old—a goal too easily attainable. Consider the examples of Jimi Hendrix, Jim Morrison, Kurt Cobain, and Tupac Shakur. While considered difficult and rebellious in life, all are perfect profit machines in death. They are now young for eternity. Their beauty will never fade. They are role models that advertise the virtues of going down in flames at a young age. These rebels to the death sound antisocial, but maybe they are just what the capitalists called for.

Why would ruling-class cabals promote martyr artists and products carrying the naïve, nihilistic, and seemingly antisocial messages of doomed youth? Well, we have rampant unemployment and high taxes. Why? We have too many workers. We wouldn't have to pay all this unemployment and all these pensions if these workers would do us a favor and die younger. And as Wyndham Lewis wrote in *The Doom of Youth* (1932):

> ...on top of everything else, a man actually has the effrontery to expect more and more, the older he gets. That is the last straw! For doing exactly the same thing, only not quite so efficiently...

It is in the interest of big business for there to be fewer workers and for them to have shorter lives, and it would be great if they didn't reproduce either. Oh, and shouldn't we eliminate those alpha-male types who start unions and revolutions? Nip them in the bud! Creating cults of self-destruction is a great way to cull the herd of its most potentially troublesome alphas. Encourage them to live dangerously and self-immolate by means of hot rods to hell, extreme sports, drive-by shooting, binge boozing, and glamorized narcotics. Whereas once it was the weak and sickly youth who were disposed of by banishment or exposure, the consumer society now shows a preference for their survival—we need cogs and drones now, not heroes. So the rock-and-roll genocide of robust, restive, and revolutionary youth has replaced the traditional disposal by war.

Do the math. The American Civil War caused 620,000 deaths; the First World War 116,703; the Second World War 407,316; Korea 36,576; and Vietnam 58,207. As of this writing, the Iraq war, officially over in its eighth year, has accounted for 4,427 deaths (though nearly 32,000 wounded); the war in Afghanistan, now in its tenth year, has caused "only" 1,357 American fatalities. War just isn't what it was. Obviously our rulers need alternative means of liquidating the warrior stock. They need to remind the young bucks to live dangerously and give them the means to off themselves because, after all, the good die young, leaving a good-looking corpse and possibly royalties.

Increasing the supply of drugs and guns eventually controlled the black ghettos that had rioted in the sixties. The same method seems to work well with artists, intellectuals, and other troublemakers. Give them heroin and guns and guitars, and for God's sake, keep them downtown! As long as natural leaders are neutralized, as long as the young can be alienated from the old, and as long as women and men can be set at one another's throats, it is unlikely that anyone will pay much attention to the more essential issues of ethics and social justice. But first off, let's make men into permanent boys.

The contemporary casual dress movement in business is a ploy designed to disguise hierarchy and power and de-emphasize the traditional role of seniority. Casual offices tell us that it is better to dress as a boy than as a man. After all, isn't the boy stronger, more energetic, and more beautiful? And he has more of a future as a customer, so shouldn't we all be boys? And if we can't, wouldn't we be better off dead?

Youth culture tells us that we can't trust anyone over thirty and so we should die before we get old. (Hey, this could solve the social-security funding issue.) Make maturity so unappealing, so out of fashion that the survivors lose the will to live. If you don't believe me, page through men's fashion magazines and you'll see bold inversion flaunted, even in the advertising: wimps, nerds, dweebs, sissies, nancy boys, and mincing weenies cavorting in adult boy clothes. These are permanent beta boys who have abjured manhood for a life on the edge of gender in a sartorial neverland.

Fashion is for followers, and the man of fashion is now a Peter Pan who will never grow up any more than is absolutely necessary. The male in fashion is not your father, but he is very much his mother's son. He is a good boy, a good companion to women, and a fine, tractable employee. We learned back in the nineteenth century that children could do well at factory work; apparently, they are still doing it well in parts of Asia. The boy/man is well suited to the tasks of the drone. He is unlikely to be supporting a family. And should he settle down, it will likely be a DINK situation (double income, no kids).

The men of fashion are youth-worshipping gays and the metrosexuals. Fashion's men will desperately attempt to prolong their youth well beyond the range of their less-well-off peers. They will not only have their appearance radically altered by cosmetic docs, but they can also sport the fashions of the age snob and affect a rock-and-roll sensibility to accompany it. If they can no longer be young themselves, then they can attempt to form an entourage of youth or, failing that, quietly off themselves.

But I will not go so quickly or quietly. I am going to get very old and enjoy it immensely, and in doing so, I and my graying rakehell accomplices will turn the clock back to the way things used to be—the way they ought to be. We've got to live like kings or die trying!

For the world to change for the better, or indeed survive, we must embrace age and fight the phony youth-god fashion. The man who is well past youth and any hope of presenting himself as a facsimile thereof can take comfort in the fact that he is not alone. The now ironically termed baby boomers are a huge bloc of unfashionable age. They are divided between those who would be as young as possible by any means necessary and those who find some satisfaction in accepting their natural state. I'm old and I'm loving it!

Although there are signs that youth may become bored with worshipping itself, it is still important to try to avoid being considered over the hill. I have found certain things discourage that conclusion; for example, a sharp wit, an encyclopedic knowledge of popular music, or the possession of good marijuana. Young people also respect wealth, real estate, exceptional decor, facial hair, wine, art and other collections, criminal records, ability at cards and games such as pool and Ping-Pong, and knowledge of ancient bohemian movements. Ancient history should only be recounted for the young at their insistence. But expertise is ours to give. Here, son, let me show you how to mix that drink.

Just say no to youth. Let's get old and enjoy the hell out of it. Let's make maturity cool again. It is time to bring back the suit, the tie, and the hat as emblems of manhood. Manhood is the goal, and youth graduates to manhood through rites of passage. Adopting this important element of warrior societies would help us erase the decadent youth worship of pop culture. I suggest that a nondenominational form of the bar mitzvah be adopted universally. Youth should be rewarded and recognized for officially reaching manhood, perhaps by being ritually presented with a suit with long trousers, a fedora, and a wristwatch.

The beards that are now in fashion, evoking Che Guevara, ZZ Top, or Rutherford B. Hayes, seem to be a step in the right direction. These present man as a natural man, a manly man, fit for the graying revolutionary vanguard.

Age must make youth come to it. Attempts by older persons to court or imitate their juniors can only be regarded as pathetic. It is far better to be an aloof, unrestored, even half-dilapidated, genuine antique than one that is a refinished or trendily slipcovered youth pretender. But should you find yourself mocked or chided by foolish youth, you can always point out the obvious: youth is not an exclusive club. Everyone is young once, but not everyone is intelligent or talented. Youths can't deny it; they won't be young for long, whereas there is a decent chance that I will be quoted forever.

Wyndham Lewis concluded *The Doom of Youth* thus:

I prophesy that two centuries hence a long and sweeping snow white beard will be an emblem of aristocratic privilege...the supreme token that the person possessing it belongs to the ruling class—that he is a member of that superclass who do not die, like dogs, after ten years of an active life.

Just remember, youth is a dead end. Maturity is the future. What we need is a total reintegration of society from top to bottom. That seems extraordinarily unlikely, but if we start it as a fad or fashion, perhaps no one will notice it's serious until it's too late to stop manhood from coming back. We men must start acting like men again. Wear vested suits, white shirts, and ties, smoke pipes, drive station wagons, drink Manhattans, and call the wife "honey." In short, grow up. If necessary I will wear a Homburg and monocle and stroll with a cane to make my point. The future hangs in the balance.

HOW TO RESIST
THE SYMPTOMS OF SENILITY

They say these days that sixty is the new forty. This is clearly not true in the Midwest, but generally older men are more youthful than ever. In part this is due to better medical care, diet, and exercise, but it is also out of terror in the face of the youth culture that we ourselves spearheaded decades ago. I never felt better in my life, personally.

The secret of prolonged vitality is to "lively up yourself and don't be no drag," as Bob Marley put it. W. B. Yeats wrote: "An aged man is but a paltry thing / A tattered coat upon a stick, unless / Soul clap its hands and sing, and louder sing / For every tatter in its mortal dress…" Clapping and singing are good. As are dancing and sports. All my friends over forty who play hoops have had knee operations, but there's no shame in golf and croquet, that most vicious of games, which makes up in cruelty what it lacks in exertion.

Scientists note that seniors who play bridge and do crossword puzzles are less likely to suffer from dementia, but whether this is because they play or that they play because they don't have incipient dementia, who knows?

Either way, it's good to keep yourself sharp enough to tear opponents to shreds, at least verbally.

Today an astonishing number of men seek to conceal their age by dyeing their hair. Eventually every dyer is going to look too old for his painted hair; he may even suddenly find himself ridiculous. It's better to have a face that's too young for the gray than too old for the brown. You can't suddenly transition from dyed jet black to white unless you shave your head, and even then, your psyche may be bruised and your reputation tarnished. I'm waiting to see how Bob Costas handles this.

Andy Warhol's adoption of the silver wig by his early forties was brilliant. He realized that white hair combined with a youthful face takes one out of the realm of chronological age and into a realm of mythical age. Warhol also lied about his age but never spectacularly. He would simply make himself out a few years older or younger than he was, not aiming to create a specific idea of his age but rather a lack of surety; since the sources would always be contradictory, there would be no fact. If you are listed on social networks, why not give several different dates of birth? Not only will you have more than one choice of age, you can celebrate multiple birthdays.

As you move inexorable toward extinction, you will look like less of a fool if you take care of your body; lean and limber muscles can be held on to for quite a long time. Other organs, such as the memory, are harder to exercise. This is where a few simple mnemonic tricks may ameliorate the memory banks. My own memory has lost a step over the years and the data has overflowed its vessel. Living in a megalopolis, one becomes acquainted with a great many people. Most are soon forgotten, but should they remember you, there's the rub. You will likely be considered a snob instead of the pre-senile overtaxed citizen that you are, but even that has its uses.

Recently I was attending an art exhibition where a friendly German dealer took me aside to discuss his wares. In the course of conversation, he asked me if my wife were my daughter. "Yes," I said, "but we sleep together." He began to blink rapidly and decided to change the subject, gesturing toward a large rotating angular mirror. "It makes you dizzy, no?" he said. "No," I replied. "Maybe because of my astronaut training."

My wife is twenty years my junior. There is no generation gap. We are both adults. It works. Men are sometimes emotionally younger than women. I think it was Nietzsche who said that the average forty-eight-year-old woman is more mature than any man.

Why would a young woman want an older man? Well, ask one. But if you ask me, we are smarter, wiser, better at sex yet less likely to fuck around and dump them, and we have more dough so they can make us pay if we do. We are also probably more stable and have better stories.

When my nine-year-old son talks about his future wife, I tell him, "She probably hasn't been born yet." Trans-generational mating is an ancient and natural state of affairs, and I find it strange that anyone would suspect my wife of being my daughter. Certainly I could have a daughter my wife's age, and if I did, I might have recruited her mother's successor from among her friends. You may think that strange, but consider the fact that nature empowers men to reproduce until far later in life than women (and we get bitter later too). Younger women also have sharp memories.

At a certain point, when one has reached acquaintance overload, it is necessary to forget someone in order to later recall someone new. My best mnemonic device is my wife. Her memory chips are not yet full, and she can often prompt me as to just who this long-lost friend is who remembers our last conversation in depth. In ancient Rome, those who were involved in the public life often had servants with excellent memories accompany them, whispering in their ears the names of those who approached them. Today young personal assistants still perform this task for politicians and magazine editors. Some powerful persons even wear earpieces at public events, through which spotter assistants can remind them of the identity of their interlocutors.

Not having this luxury, I simply adopted a strategy of smiling and greeting as a long-lost bosom buddy anyone who approaches me in a manner suggesting prior familiarity. "Hi!" I'll say, beaming with delight. I have found that the name issue often doesn't come up if your first remark is "You look fantastic!" This not only suggests remembrance to the stranger, but it serves as a wonderful distraction. This strategy fails only when you have never actually met the person and they were accosting you on sheer nerve.

Should you find yourself in the awkward situation of forgetting the name attached to a familiar face and you are with an escort, inform the latter that, should you pause, he or she must introduce him- or herself immediately, forcing the bogey to introduce him- or herself, so that your forgetfulness or obliviousness will not be discovered.

HOW TO AIL

"I don't know much about medicine, but I know what I like."

—S. J. Perelman

No matter how healthy we are, we are likely to fall sick once in a while. We live at peril in a dog-eat-dog world, an eat-or-be-eaten universe. Our air and water are poisoned by industry, and most food is an unreasonable facsimile of what humans thrive on. Germs festering in the unhealthy populace nibble away at us, alien fungi set up shop on our persons; strange viruses invade our cells, parasitically altering our evolutionary equilibrium.

But this is not always a bad thing. Even a germ may have some wisdom to impart. And feeling awful can be good for our general perspective. You don't really know how good you usually feel until you feel awful.

Generally speaking, one desires to recover from illness, unless of course to continue on living would constitute a "fate worse than death."

Therefore the best approach to sickness is usually recovery, although sometimes we may wish to linger in our indolent sequestering for a while before putting our symptoms aside as a complete recovery is effected (or affected). We may wish to languish abed, enjoying the concerned ministrations of others while ignoring our quotidian duties. We may have drudgery that we prefer to postpone or palm off on another, and nothing provides a better cover for the shirker than illness, as we tend to learn in elementary school.

The best cure for many illnesses is bed rest, which provides plenty of opportunities to catch up on one's reading and movie watching. Sometimes having a respiratory problem can give a smoker a good head start on kicking the habit, and similarly, a few days in bed can work wonders for the livers of the cocktail addicted.

Trying to work through sickness is a bad idea. Especially when you show up at the job and cough all over the workforce. If you're under the weather, stay home. You're probably there too little as it is. Enjoy your bed, your books, and your backlog of unwatched Criterion DVDs, and allow anyone who happens to be devoted to you to indulge your afflicted whimsicality.

But after an illness has mostly run its course and boredom with convalescence has begun to set in, it's time for healing to begin. Despite what most doctors and other authorities will tell you, a good patient takes charge of his own cures and recoveries. Doctors are not priests or miracle workers. They make mistakes frequently, as their insurance premiums attest. Physicians may be preoccupied with marital problems or their golf swings, and crucial symptoms may escape their notice. Although their fees and demeanor would suggest otherwise, they are eminently fallible. So whether you let on or not, take charge of your own case. You'll be glad you did.

If you watch television while recuperating you will notice that a great many commercials are attempting to sell us pharmaceuticals, and if we are treated by an American MD, he is likely to try out these potions on us, if only because the pharmaceutical companies will be more likely to send him to Tulum or Maui if he writes enough prescriptions. Notice that most of these medicines have stated side effects that are considerably worse than the consequences of the disease they purport to cure—side effects such as death. Do not be eager to consume these drugs, as the prescriber himself may have no idea as to their mechanism or likely effect. Most doctors, intimidated by rigid professional standards and uninterested in empirical evidence, work by rote. You may be prescribed powerful antibiotics for viral illnesses against which they are useless, or given large doses of hepatotoxic acetaminophen and told to call in the morning (should you survive). Remember that if you do nothing but rest and eat well, chances are you'll recover anyway, without giving your doctor a chance to kill you.

Before you turn your case over to a physician, have a good look at the physician. How is his health? Is he morbidly obese? Does he drink too much? (Most doctors will tell you that you are drinking too much if you drink more than they do.) Does he look old for his age? Is he a rotten son of a bitch? Does he possibly envy you? Be careful, as these croakers have the power of life and death, which often leads them to confuse themselves with deities.

There are also the worlds of alternative medicine and homeopathy, which may or may not prove more effective than conventional medicine but are certainly more fun to talk about. In any case, homeopathy is less likely to poison the patient than our allopathic network of science-fiction cure cartels. My advice is to try to get a good-looking French female doctor to come see you, or a good acupuncturist, and make sure you get lots of liquids including a glass of red with meals. If she prescribes an enema, don't reject it out of hand. You may be full of shit. And if she brings out the leeches, be sure to get it on film.

Recovery can be easy, especially if you are not particularly ill. As we have often been told, an ounce of prevention equals a pound of cure, so taking to your bed before an illness fully asserts itself is the best policy. It is the simplest form of preventive medicine. Go to bed; catch up on your sleep and your novel-reading schedule. There's nothing more irritating than someone showing up for work coughing, sneezing, and sniveling, spreading viruses and bacteria throughout the workplace. Not only is working sick harmful to yourself, but it is also a threat to others who would be well served by your involuntary commitment to a medical facility or, at the very least, your banishment from the place of business. Take to bed with books. I would suggest Sax Rohmer's series of novels about the insidious Dr. Fu Manchu; they will make you feel better about not consulting a doctor.

On calling in sick, one should insist that the only reason for your absence is a concern for the well-being of your fellows. "I would come in, but I don't want anyone else to catch this dreadful bug." Coughing, sneezing into the telephone, and speaking in a hoarse, practically unrecognizable voice will not only help your case but also make your co-workers appreciate your absence all the more. Just be certain that you return to the job before your superiors notice that things are humming along fine without you.

Taking to your bed should be done in style. Make sure the bed is made with fresh linens, with plenty of extra pillows and blankets available. You will undoubtedly want to prop yourself up to read and watch films, and, in the latter, less contagious phase, receive well-wishers and volunteer caregivers. Put on your best pajamas and have a good robe and slippers available for trips to the bathroom and little exercise forays around the house. Good pajamas help one to maintain a will to live. And should you find yourself hospitalized, good pajamas and robes can make the difference between life and death. As a signifier of socioeconomic status, fine pajamas (as opposed to some tattered hospital gown) will put professional caregivers and other hospital personnel on alert that you are a person of importance who is likely to bring a significant malpractice suit to bear in case of mistreatment. If a specialist is coming in to see you, put on a smoking jacket first.

As the squeaky wheel gets the grease, the pain-in-the-ass patient will inevitably enjoy more attention from doctors and nurses. A good case study of ruses and rhetoric for the convalescent is the behavior of Sheridan Whiteside (played by Monty Woolley) in *The Man Who Came to Dinner*. And don't let yourself be brainwashed by the term "patient." Do you know what it means, for God's sake? It comes from the Latin for "sufferer" and means "bearing or enduring [evil of any kind] with composure." Fuck that! Your life isn't the book of Job! Be impatient. Be demanding. Generally patients are conditioned by the system to be patient, to wait, and to have low expectations of their caregivers, who are in turn conditioned to be gruff, uncaring, and condescending. Study Whiteside's lines, such as "Go in and read the life of Florence Nightingale and learn how unfitted you are for your chosen profession."

The next chapter deals with the problem of doctors and their attitudes, but by all means question the quack. Do not simply accept his diagnosis and course of treatment, but have it explained to your complete satisfaction. He may have overlooked vital information that you possess. Do you know how many doctors operate on the wrong knee or the wrong side of the brain? Do you know how many drinks the guy had last night? This morning?

Another tip for the hospital bound is make sure that there are plenty of visitors and, should you lack visitors or not, beautiful and expensive flowers, even if you have to send them to yourself, again serve as a conspicuous status indicator. Because hospital personnel often tend to be surly and contentious, it is a good idea to attempt discreet tipping, or bribe them with candy and other treats if they will not accept actual tips. Most patients would not even think of tipping their nurses and orderlies, which makes your gratuities even more significant. If you are worried about your condition, you might even offer a nurse private employment once you recover; this could guarantee her or his interest in your survival.

Make sure that within easy reach in one's sickroom are plenty of liquids and tissues and that there is an adequate wastebasket handy. I find in case of a phlegmfest it's good to have two wastebaskets, one nearby and one for three-point attempts.

I always have a broad selection of good books on hand just in case influenza strikes. The classics make for particularly good reading when one is ill because they don't remind you of work or current events and often there is a lot of brutal warfare and one can fantasize about one's co-workers or competitors in the roles of the losers—such as Pompey and Mark Antony. I also take care to regularly cut out the *New York Times* crossword on Fridays and Saturdays when I don't have time to do it. These are handy for sick days as well as long airplane rides. In the event of a more serious, mind numbing-fever, it's good to have some of the easier Wednesday and Thursday puzzles in stock as well. Even a few Mondays, in case you lapse into coma.

Chicken soup as medicine is not some Jewish myth. It is genuinely therapeutic and anodyne. Especially if it has some nice, organic, free-range white meat in it. Arrange for a friend to provide chicken soup. They say feed a cold and starve a fever, but I find sick days an excellent opportunity to lose weight, so if you don't have a fever, pretend. Loss of appetite will also help you gain sympathy from significant others. And your return to work will be more dramatic should you appear to have wasted slightly.

You may be tempted to work while laid up. This is a noble instinct but don't tax yourself. You need all your strength in reserve for healing. If you must work, try limiting yourself to pencil and paper (small pieces) at brief intervals. Having a computer handy could be unwise as it may tempt you to look up your symptoms on the Internet, which leads only to psychosomatic complications or cheating on the crossword. I also advise avoiding such entertainments as *House M.D., ER, Grey's Anatomy, Scrubs*, et al. If you watch *House M.D.*, no matter what your symptoms, you will visualize your innards in animated shutdown, get worse, and become convinced you have lupus or a tiny twin trapped in your scrotum.

Do not return to work until your symptoms have vanished completely, but on your return to work, do not rush into your usual routine hastily lest your vigor be interpreted as guilt over your absence. Pace yourself. Leave early for a few days after announcing with minimal pep that you are not quite yourself. Otherwise your co-workers may think you are showing off.

Should you be lucky enough to get laryngitis, you might develop a temporarily sexy voice. Don't fail to take advantage of this condition to record messages for your answering machine or to telephone attractive persons who have flirted with you recently.

Sickness, within reason, is a luxury. It is an involuntary vacation that provides an opportunity for rest and meditation. For compulsive workers, it can serve as a wake-up call to one's fellow workers as to just how dependent on you they are. (Although if you've been coasting, it can have the opposite effect.) It's nature's way of telling us to slow down. And as with slow food and languid sex, unhurried medicine is usually a good idea.

While sick days may provide a refreshing supplement to our vacation and personal days, nobody wants to hear about your illness, or any of your other problems, for that matter. As the Duke of Bedford wrote in his *Book of Snobs*:

Do not talk about health; that is definitely out… No one is ever interested in your health, whether you have been ill or as fit as a fiddle. Everybody is interested only in himself.

ON DEALING
WITH DOCTORS

"Yesterday the doctor told me to stop drinking. I woke up this morning and I was the doctor."

—Tom Waits

It is not uncommon for professionals, particularly those who exhibit diplomas, to be guilty of arrogance and hubris. Doctors make a practice of keeping clients waiting, hence "waiting rooms," while other trades seem to be able to keep to a schedule that is more of a two-way street. Is the waiting room simply a device intended to put the patient in his place, making him grateful for a few minutes of the doctor's precious time?

Years ago I broke an ankle and was treated by a doctor who prided himself on healing the bones of millionaire athletes. On a follow-up visit, I was kept waiting for two hours with no explanation. When the white-coated doctor entered the examination room, he took up a set of X-rays, examined them, and proclaimed "God, I'm good!" Moving inside his discomfort zone, I informed him that whatever his mechanical skills, his blithely imperious attitude was ungentlemanly and unacceptable and that I would never wait for him again. Remarkably, it seemed that no one had ever complained about this before, and I received an actual apology.

Most of us have few friends who are doctors. One reason is that doctors stick together so they don't have to give us free advice. And like cops, they have each other's back. It's really them against us. Doctors are often full of shit, but it's not all their fault, as they have been rigorously trained to be full of shit. And even the noblest and most altruistic of croakers has been brain-washed to go by the book, a book written in committee and in consort with pharmaceutical cartels. But this orthodoxy has weakened doctors' powers of observation and deduction over the years, so even if we manage to find a good doctor, we have to use strategy and rhetoric to make sure that we are treated right.

The first rule of seeking medical treatment is: don't take any shit.

Recently, I went to a dermatologist to have my fair skin checked for time-bomb actinic keratoses, a leading cause of death among golfers, and to get my annual lecture on using sunscreen. Having jumped through hoops to get a referral—including a visit to the new primary-care doctor who looked like Burt Ward, Batman's original Robin—I had my insurance card in my hand and a referral on file. Arriving at the desk, I had to wait two or three minutes while the receptionists finished a gossip session, and then they greeted me as one might greet an unwanted beggar. I was told to hand over my card, again fill out the questionnaire already on file (though no data had changed), and give them my referral. I replied that the referral was on file, but apparently the older gossiping receptionist had not entered my insurance codes properly and now she couldn't find it. She petulantly insisted that there was no referral. Since I had spent hours locating and securing a primary care doctor, then visited that doctor, secured a referral for this visit, and taken a $20 taxi ride seventy-five blocks uptown, I was annoyed.

I said, "So what am I supposed to do now, go home?" Perhaps my tone was a little hard, as the senior member of the reception team, no doubt used to the humble acquiescence of cowed patients, was startled and uttered, "Oh, my God!" in a tone that would have been appropriate if I had just pulled an AK-47 on them. The older woman froze, but the fact that I was furiously keying an outraged e-mail into my BlackBerry seemed to motivate the younger receptionist to retrace her steps and she soon managed to locate my referral on their computer. It was interesting that simply reacting to their

habitual condescending manner was enough to shock them and shake
them into action. They seemed genuinely nervous. Was I the first patient
who was not afraid of them?

I believe that the thrall in which patients are held by the medical and
insurance industries, the relentless corporate antagonism, begins with
this sort of personal intimidation. Patients are there because there is
something wrong with them. They are sick and tired, often old and confused, and generally as fearful of a hostile, impenetrable bureaucracy as they
are of pain and death. I tried to recall the last time I had seen medical desk
personnel treat their unfortunate charges with consideration, but I came
up blank. Why they don't take mug shots and fingerprints of patients
escapes me.

Hostility, generally aimed at the helpless and powerless, is a tone set by
doctors, who tend to treat their patients as idiots, showing them less
compassion than the average practitioner of veterinary medicine. They're
still doing the old "white man's burden" routine.

How many times have I heard something like: "Hello, Glenn, I'm
Doctor Smith." This immediately positions the doctor as sahib and the
patient as untouchable, and so it must be corrected immediately. I can reply,
"Hello, Doctor Smith, I'm *Mister* O'Brien." But it's possible that the physician will fail to notice this subtlety, so you should be prepared to use his first
name next. If that doesn't work, you can always resort to calling him "pal,"
"buddy," "chief," or "boss," which is probably the preferred derisive honorific
of our time.

You are not being rude, rather you are correcting him and bringing him
down to earth, where diseases exist. By restoring a proper on-the-level relationship between doctor and patient you may, in fact, prevent malpractice
through carelessness. The less you kowtow to a doctor, the more care he will
take with you. If somehow you can manage to convince him that you are
his equal, he may even take an interest in your case.

Receptionists and assistants usually take their cues in arrogance from the physicians who employ them, but their attitudes are compounded by the tone set by HMOs, the medical insurance providers who dominate health care in the United States. Employees of HMOs more closely resemble attorneys than medical workers because their primary mission is denying clients their rightful benefits.

The weakness of HMOs and other bureaucracies is that they are not monolithic. Their best agents are remarkably efficient in denying coverage, confusing clients, and generally dissuading them from seeking further treatment, but not all customer-service people are equally ruthless. By pursuing a policy of tirelessly moving on to the next agent and then the next, one will invariably wind up speaking to someone with humane tendencies. Do not give up. Move up the flowchart until you encounter someone with whom charm, reason, and persistence may stand a chance. Just remember, the things that irritate you will irritate those paid to deal with you.

Decorum will get you many places, but it will get you nowhere in a hospital or a doctor's office. If you are not being treated right or even treated at all, why not scream? Not just a little venting of steam but a real blood-curdling, ululating scream from the depths of Hell. Primal, as they used to say. The point is to horrify and frighten everyone within earshot. Become an issue of control. As soon as you have issued a good feral caterwaul at high volume, you are in control. Suddenly you will be listened to. Waited on. Humored. You will have challenged their authority by creating a scene, but it's your scene and they will have to play along. They will all urgently hope that you do not scream again, and they will understand why you did it. They may even respect your nerve. But they will shut you up by serving you.

In a medical establishment, unless you have endowed it, you are swimming upstream. You must be prepared to use rhetoric, tactics, and showmanship. Remember the slogan of our species, the principle that got us to the top of the evolutionary heap: survival of the fittest. Don't hesitate to have a fit.

HOW TO EXIT

If you have spent much time in Florida, you have probably noticed that death isn't what it used to be. Today millions of people have successfully eluded the Reaper's scythe long after their historical expiration or sell-by date. We have large communities of blonde octogenarian widows in bare-midriff outfits surviving far beyond their utility. We have retiree security guards with walkers. We have squadrons of wheeled humans tooling around malls in oxygen masks. The would-be dead are alive. Lively, even!

There are many factors involved in this, including the advances of modern medicine, relative peace, and the destruction of natural enemies in the habitat. I also suspect stubbornness and revenge as motivators. I think many of the aged live on mostly to wreak vengeance on their children or former spouses. Even widows may persist in life, spurred on by the fact that their revenge will be incomplete if his fortune remains unspent.

But observing the aged closely will inevitably lead one to the realization that life isn't all it's cracked up to be. It is undoubtedly better to go out on top, while one is in reasonable possession of his faculties, than to stretch existence out until one becomes a caricature of one's former self. A study of the mutations perpetrated under the rubric of cosmetic medicine should be enough to convince any reasonable person that there are far worse fates than death. Of course, in practice it's hard to decide exactly when is the optimum moment for extinction. Generally speaking, a good rule of thumb is: are you still having fun?

But we must, by all means, avoid the indignities of having our last view of this earthly realm take place in a drab, fluorescent-lit hospital among the ghouls and zombies who inhabit the medical profession and their grotesque charges, or to have our consciousness impinged upon by pharmaceuticals that will impair our control during the crucial denouement of our personal drama. Death is not an abnormal function, and it should be negotiated with style, hopefully in a manner consistent with the best passages of our lives.

In other words, if you have retained any choice in the matter, go home if you sense the end coming on. Take to your bed, unless you have a particularly comfortable and picturesque favorite chair; however, it's best if you can recline sufficiently so that you will not strike the floor awkwardly upon the departure of the spirit.

As J. P. Donleavy so eloquently put it: "Dismiss from your mind as an asshole anyone who tells you you can have a happy death." Living is what we are made for, so death is undoubtedly going to disappoint. We may not even be good at it. But we must put on a good front because hopefully we have a legacy to entrust to our loved ones, if not to the race in general. In other words, this is one of those instances where we're just going to have to make the best of it.

The first rule is to banish from your presence any miserable bastard who might try to upstage you at the penultimate moment, in other words, the clergy. Should you find yourself surrounded by unwelcome folk, remember that dying words are accorded a certain gravity in our society, so any curses or imprecations you may utter now will be taken more seriously than usual. Try "Get out!" or "I'll see you in Hell!" and see if that doesn't clear the room of loiterers making a last-ditch attempt to crash your last will and testament.

By this point we hope you will have found a physician who will accommodate you with the anodynes of your preference. A nice dose of morphine, a martini (in drip form, if necessary), perhaps a cigar, or even a hit of crack procured from the pool boy will help you achieve a cheerful and relatively pain-free liftoff. At this point a doctor has no excuse not to accede to your wishes; there is no risk of addiction.

If time permits, give some thought to your last words. If you can come up with something memorable, it will certainly survive you and enhance your reputation even after it's out of your hands. A good line can comfort bereaved loved ones—and it is our last opportunity to make others jealous or even haunt all their days with remorse.

Lord Byron's "Good night" is classic. Aleister Crowley's "I am perplexed" was a good one. As was Tallulah Bankhead's "Codeine...bourbon..." And Joan Crawford's "Don't you dare ask God to help me." And Wyndham Lewis's "Mind your own business!" If anyone has topped Douglas Fairbanks Sr.'s "I've never felt better," I suppose it would be Vespasian with "I think I am turning into a god." Or Oscar Wilde, who said, "Either that wallpaper goes, or I do."

If you have any serious unfinished business, don't forget the dying declaration, which, even though it is considered hearsay, is admissible in court. If you have neglected an opportunity to "drop a dime" on an enemy, this is your last but possibly your best opportunity.

There is a low opinion of suicide in contemporary society, which stems from the ambition of the state and the church to control the most basic conditions of our lives, such as our very existence. But as many noble Romans and Greeks proved, it can be a better option in certain situations— as when one is surrounded by vicious and implacable enemies who can't wait to display your head on a pike, a situation comparable to that of many terminally ill persons who are kept alive in discomfort for billing purposes masquerading as ethics.

Falling on one's sword was the traditional Roman method for the besieged soldier and it certainly left a more presentable corpse than Hemingway's shotgun did, but it requires a certain handiness and balance that we may lack. The best exits are usually those for which the intention to perish is somewhat shrouded in adventurous enterprise. Say, before the Feds arrive one is seized by the urge to take the schooner out one last time just as Hurricane Zelda bears down on the coast, or one is overtaken by a sudden interest in hot-air ballooning from Guam to Easter Island.

Should the government have neglected to seize your entire estate, it is important that your last will and testament be drawn up by competent lawyers who are entirely on your team. Otherwise, should Hell have cable, you might learn that your property has fallen into the hands of your archenemy or least favorite ex-wife. Don't leave a dry and boring will, all legalese. Liven it up with unexpurgated commentary on your contemporaries while taking care not to raise a red flag on the "being of sound mind" clause.

As to the final resting place of one's remains, there is some comfort in installing them in a scenic location rather than dumping them into the sea, where they might wind up floating amid all those six-pack rings and plastic bottles in the mid-Pacific, or scattering them to the winds, where they might wind up in the drain of a car wash. Having a gravesite, whether it holds your ashes in a can or your bones in a box, will give your fans a place to gather; just choose your spot carefully, with an eye to possible eminent-domain issues in the future.

I haven't made any final determination on what to do with my leftovers. Sometimes I think it's better to be burned first, in the manner of the Greek heroes, and so avoid becoming worm fodder. But maybe worm fodder is the green way to go, buried in a simple pine box. Those burial vaults are creepy, hermetically sealed, Pharaonic capsules apparently designed to prevent one's carbon from reentering the biosphere until Jesus intervenes. Sorry, I want my molecules back in food-chain circulation immediately. It looks stuffy in there. I'd rather be compost.

IMMORTALITY:
WHAT TO DO LATER

According to a poll by ABC News, eighty-nine percent of Americans believe in Heaven and think that they are probably going to end up there. Most believe that Paradise will house their spirit only, although the resurrection of the body is old Christian doctrine and part of the Roman Catholic creed. Among Americans it is mostly very religious Protestants, the demographic that also tends to see Heaven as Christians only, who believe that their meat puppets will rejoin them in the future when Jesus makes his encore.

A smaller percentage of the populace believes in the existence of Hell, only fifty-nine percent according to a 2008 Pew Forum survey (down from seventy-one percent in a 2001 Gallup poll). The Catholic Church also preaches the existence of Purgatory, where those not sufficiently pure for Heaven will suffer temporal punishment until their sins are cleansed. For centuries this tenet was a tremendous source of revenue for the Church in the form of indulgence marketing. The Roman Catholic Church also posited the existence of a fourth state of afterlife known as Limbo, where the unbaptized reside until the Last Judgment. Actually there have been two Limbos. The Limbo of the Fathers was where Old Testament patriarchs resided until Christ "descended into Hell" and opened the gates of Heaven to them. Then there was the Limbo of Infants (which has been considerably de-emphasized in recent years), where the souls of dead, unbaptized infants are held; their ultimate fate remains unspecified.

The current pope, Benedict XVI, authorized the publication *The*

Hope of Salvation for Infants Who Die Without Being Baptized. Authored by the Pope's think tank, the International Theological Commission, it holds out some hope that the unbaptized will eventually enjoy the beatific vision. Church authorities have denied, however, that the current Pope has "closed Limbo." Still, the specifics of even Heaven and Hell have become very sketchy.

Culturally we still seem to be living with a sort of Dante's *Inferno* view of Hell, while Heaven remains a mix of Renaissance paintings of angelic aerial maneuvers around God's throne and *New Yorker* cartoons with clouds, harps, and halos. With 3-D production taking over Hollywood, a new model of the afterlife is overdue. Heaven will probably look a lot like the saccharine 1998 Robin Williams vehicle *What Dreams May Come*, and Hell like the wretched John Cusack vehicle *2012*.

But more and more of us are abandoning traditional Christian scenarios and going Far Eastern on the issue, taking up with enthusiasm the reincarnation beliefs of Buddhists and Hindus. I think it's hard for hedonists to imagine bliss without a body. For some reason, Americans and Europeans who become interested in their cycles of incarnation generally find that they were Egyptian royals. But try as we might, we tend to wind up facing the facts that we just don't know what, if anything, follows the present life. And if we don't remember past lives, do they really matter anyway?

Personally I'm hoping for reincarnation in a good-looking body, but I'm not holding my breath. There isn't much one can do to prepare for a possible afterlife, aside from entering the void with an open mind and a cheerful disposition. Attachment to a world in which circumstances will not allow us to remain can only spoil our enjoyment of experiences to come, if any.

The best we can do is to make ourselves immortal the American way—incorporate. Our flesh may shrivel and die, but our corporate beings can last...well, forever-ish. We can't all be Fords, or Edisons, or

Jack Daniels, but hopefully we can leave something behind—a stack of books, a company, maybe a dynasty. And hopefully what we have left behind will continue to enrich the world and enrich our family, friends, and well-wishers. Who knows? Maybe we will ourselves move on to some reward or punishment and find amusing companionship among the blessed we encounter, or the damned, as the case may be. But if we are extinguished, at least, we have left behind something of a fan club of family, friends, and well-wishers and moved on.

Should you find yourself floating above your prone body, hovering somewhere around the ceiling of your boudoir or hospital bed, you may be on the way out of this present sphere. This is no time to panic. It happens to everyone. We have all heard stories of "going toward the light," and undoubtedly in such circumstances one has little to lose by following the conventional wisdom. However, perusal of the Egyptian and Tibetan books of the dead, as well as the traditions of Greek mystery cults, provides certain clues that might help. If the light happens to be accompanied by noxious smoke, it's best not to go in that direction. You might wind up right back where you started. Or in Detroit.

Should you find yourself before the Halls of Judgment, the best policy is probably to follow the advice of Orpheus as channeled by Robert Graves: Avoid drinking from the black spring on the left, which is Forgetfulness; go to the clear, goldfish-stocked fountain on the right guarded by the big snake—that's Memory—and tell them that you're very thirsty and Persephone sent you.

And if that doesn't work, tell them Groucho sent you.

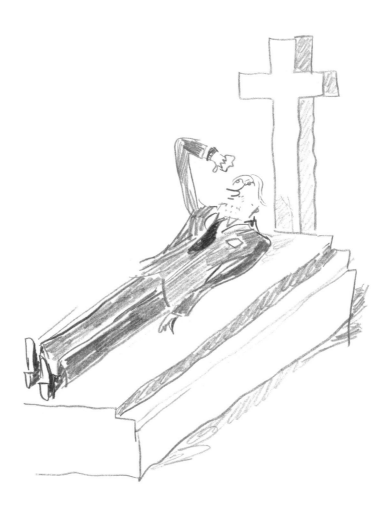

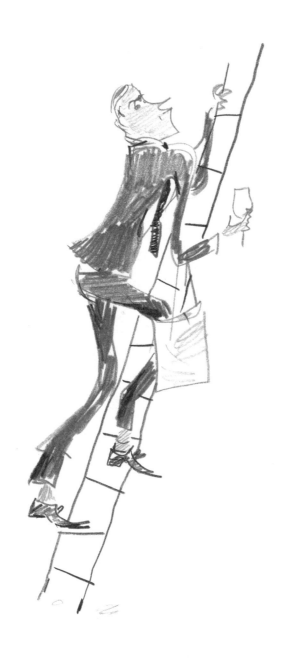

RANDOM TIPS
FOR LIVING

- When someone calls you "friend," chances are they aren't. Look for the exit. When I am referred to as "boss," or the more retro "chief," "buddy," or "pal," I feel underlying class hostility. But to address a member of the working class as "sir" is to give him dignity as a man as well as invoking centuries of persons of the chevalier class being so addressed. Addressing taxi drivers and public servants as "sir" and "ma'am" helps create a continuum of respect. Elevate the tone in your address.
- Addressing a man as "man" works only in a bohemian context, or it may convey a certain hostility: "Hey, man, what do you think you're doing?" Never address even the hippest chick as "man."
- "Gentlemen" is a good plural substitute for "sirs." It is especially effective with adolescents and others who might not ordinarily consider themselves gentlemen.
- "Darling" can be very disarming. Especially when addressing someone you find slightly dangerous and intimidating.
- If you haven't worn something for over a year, get rid of it. Exchange it at a thrift shop or donate it to your favorite charity. It might be out of style, but it's still tax-deductible.
- In America, salad bars are the leading cause of salmonella. Bars are for drinking.

• If your cab suddenly bursts into flames, you do not have to pay. Once you are safe, enlist help to make sure that the driver has escaped injury. Do not ask for a receipt. Tipping is optional.

• Don't think a simple "No!" will ever work on dogs or other animals. They aren't that conceptual. Don't be abstract; be specific. "Off!" "Down, boy!" "Drop it!" "No biting!" "No humping!" Like that.

• When somebody looks good, tell them. They will remember you.

• Nothing will dress up your look quicker or cheaper than a pro's shoeshine, and don't forget to tip.

• Complain sparingly. Nobody likes a whiner. The best part of war movies—except when the wimpy buddy gets shot down so the hero doesn't have to nobly forgo the hot chick—is when the hero says, "No excuse, sir!" even though he's got a million of 'em. He doesn't kvetch, as he's above it. Suck it up, soldier.

• If you must smoke a cigar, take the label off it. Cigars are for enjoying, not flaunting, and you don't want to be mistaken for a typical turbo-driving, Cognac-swilling jerkoff.

• A nitrogen-injecting doohickey will not only save you money, it will also save you from finishing every bottle of wine you open.

• For golfers: Always carry a set of clubs in your trunk. You never know when you might pass a deserted hole on a famous country club at dusk. Never take a mulligan. It's a slippery slope to expecting do-overs elsewhere. If your wife won't give you a mulligan, why should I?

• It's customary to tip the maid when you check out of a hotel. Instead, tip every day. You may get more towels and chocolates.

• Avoid restaurants with the word "old," "olde," or "auld" in the name, or any bar where ale comes by the yard.

• Praying demonstrably on an athletic field is in poor taste. Would you shoot hoops in a cathedral?

• Buy a *Star Trek* uniform in case you get called for jury duty.

• No matter how small your country house is, name it. Mine is called Bumfields.

- Never eat a hamburger at a horse or dog race.
- When naming a pet, don't forget a middle and last name. Do you know how many Dukes, Spots, and Kings are out there? You should be able to Google your dog.
- If you don't have a nickname, get one, and make sure your friends also have them. It's important for communicating secretly with intimates in top-secret moments in public. Similarly, mastery of antique slang can provide useful code. Never say "reefer" in public; instead say "muggles" or "gage."
- Take Jack Kerouac's advice, and don't be afraid to ask a woman for forgiveness.
- When negotiating a fee or a business deal, always have the other person name a figure first. It might be higher than you would have asked for. And if their figure is lower, smile and chuckle quietly. If it's way low, say "Well I might know someone who could do that."
- If you're single always have a toothbrush, still in its package, in the cabinet.
- People who are frequently late often set their watches ahead. What are they, nuts?
- "Cheers" is OK, but don't forget "Here's looking at you," "Skol," "Salud," "L'chaim," "Down the hatch," "Kampai," and "Here's mud in your eye."
- The *New York Times* crossword is a form of meditation. But doing it in pen if a pencil is available is grandstanding.
- Neighbors' vicious dogs can be handled by marinating tennis balls in a Valium solution.
- If a woman is pressuring you to marry, try watching Nickelodeon for a few mornings in a row.
- Bachelors should have at least one plant whose life depends on them. Before contemplating children, try a pet first.
- Every residence should have a good pair of dice and two decks (with jokers) of good cards. If you can play gin, hearts, or bridge, you need never be lonely. If you can play solitaire, you can wait.

- If you're with a vegetarian crowd, go with the flow.
- As an American, never address anyone as "Your Eminence," "Reverend," "Your Grace," "Your Honor," or "Your Royal Highness." That's over, baby! "Your Highness" is acceptable only for people really high on drugs. "Sir," "Ma'am," or "Madam" will usually do. Never address anyone as "Master," particularly male children. Never address anyone as "Mistress" unless she's wearing leather.
- A poll revealed that a high percentage of American men actually name their penises. The only acceptable names for a penis are Dick (in the U.K., Willie or Roger), Mr. Johnson, and Mr. President.
- Remember the words of Mick Jagger: "If you're out tonight on your bike, wear white."
- When reading the morning papers, start with the sports not the news, and the *Post* not the *Times*. This may help you make an easier transition from the dream state to productive wakefulness.
- Have money to invest? Chances are art and fine furniture won't drop 20 percent in a month.
- Those WWJD bracelets—as in "What Would Jesus Do?"—can be easily recycled as "What Would Jimbo Drink?"
- Joining Jews for Jesus nearly doubles your days off.
- A woman never gets tired of the word "Wow" directed her way.
- The card game hearts is vapid unless the ten of diamonds is worth ten points to the good.
- Never participate in chain e-mail. If you do, your eyelashes will fall out.
- Business cards don't cost much and they indicate you're a serious person. It's very hip to have a Japanese translation or Braille on the flip side. When boring people give you business cards, save them in your wallet to use as aliases when you meet other boring people.
- Cut flowers dress up an apartment. Live ones, however, are cost effective—plus, caring for plants is a good practice for caring for yourself. If your orchids die, can you be far behind?

• When a woman asks you if she looks fat, never say yes. If she's fat tell her she looks like Venus. But never say "Rubenesque." They're on to that.

• If someone cuts in front of you in line say, "*Mi scusi, siete dall'Italia?*"

• Wear a tuxedo for your ID photos.

• If you are asked to swear an oath, ask for a copy of *Theogeny* by Hesiod (eighth century B.C.E.) to swear on instead of a Bible.

• Don't try to interest women in sports or sci-fi. They have to come to it on their own.

• Keep a diary of your friends' birthdays. If you can't give everyone a present, at least you can call with greetings and check on party plans.

• It's okay to ask for a doggy bag in any restaurant. Just don't ask for a bitch bag.

• Carrying a small wine vintage chart in your wallet is useful, but you can expect freshness-dated beer to be pretty much the same from month to month.

• Before trying tranquilizers or psychiatric drugs, why not pick up a nice set of worry beads at your local Greek variety store?

• Leave the dust jackets on your hardcover books. They'll be worth a lot more in fifty years.

• English is the language of global business, but there are still some concepts that can only be expressed adequately in Yiddish. *Putz! Schlub!*

• If you're feeling sorry for yourself, don't talk about it. Instead, listen to Sinatra's *No One Cares* including "I Can't Get Started," "Just Friends," and "I'll Never Smile Again." It'll fix you right up.

• If someone has the poor taste to bring up their IQ, change the subject by mentioning your bowling average or golf handicap.

• Don't blame yourself if not everyone gets your jokes. Sometimes one is, in the words of the great B. S. Pully, "too smart for the room."

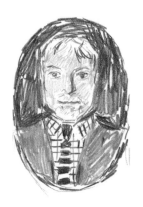

GLENN O'BRIEN: A PORTRAIT

By Jean-Philippe Delhomme

When I was first introduced to Glenn in the early 1990s, I had never met anyone like him. He was wearing a bespoke pinstripe suit and a tie that seemed straight out of a David Hockney painting. His face was half angel, half space captain, with short, silver hair and a mischievous smile.

At the time he was the creative director for the fancy department store Barneys, but what astonished me was that he did readings of his own poems for store events, poems with titles like "Beatnik Executives."

Glenn connected uptown with downtown. On one trip I saw him shake hands with John Baldessari in a gallery and have dinner with David Byrne, and when we worked on commercials together, he brought Debbie Harry and John Lurie to do the voice-overs.

When I asked older friends about Glenn, they told me about the famous music column he wrote for *Interview* magazine, which I found out later was not specifically about music. I learned that not only did Glenn work at the Factory, but Andy Warhol actually hired him as the art director for the magazine when he was still a young kid.

To add to my amazement, I discovered Glenn is a serious golfer who has played with Richard Prince and other artists and musicians. Buying the Whitney exhibition catalog on Prince shortly after, I read Glenn's long essay "The Joke of the New." Not only is he the unique art critic who can elaborate on a joke without killing it, but he also knows the right shoes to wear at the reception. I once saw him wearing luxury pajamas at Sotheby's, and sandals with socks at a fashion photography festival. The day I saw him wearing socks with sandals, I suddenly felt deadly boring wearing my Converse All Stars without socks.

When he rents a car, it's always a Lincoln town car.

He once e-mailed me that he had driven through a forest fire in Italy.

On a research trip together to L.A., he advised me to get a Beat compilation from Rhino and read Donald Barthelme, and he encouraged me to buy a pale blue polka-dot Yohji tie from Maxfield, which was the price of a suit. "Sometimes it's OK to buy an expensive tie," he said.

How does he know it all? Perhaps he has studied philosophy? A few years ago, I was reading an interview with Glenn in *Purple Fashion* magazine (where he was also modeling a kilt in a fashion story) and learned he had once been a stand-up comic and even performed at a Hell's Angels birthday party on a boat. No wonder he is totally fearless when it comes to dealing with advertising executives and fashion moguls. He has done award-winning and controversial ads for Calvin Klein, and is frequently off on shoots for Dior. I think he invented the term "Editor at Large."

In order to illustrate Glenn's column for *GQ*, "The Style Guy," I read thousands of his answers to some of the readers' strange questions, from chest-hair trimming to butt enhancement. Once I sought his words of wisdom, complaining that some new artist's career was launched in the same manner as a designer's collection. "Well, the art and fashion worlds tend to be more or less the same," he said serenely.

I could mention *TV Party*, the cult TV show he had hosted in the early 1980s, or *Downtown 81*, the poetic film he wrote about his friend Jean-Michel Basquiat.

I could mention some of his current projects, which I just heard about. But it still would be incomplete.

In fact, every time I see Glenn, I have to update his bio.

ACKNOWLEDGMENTS

Glenn O'Brien is grateful to Jean-Philippe Delhomme, Richard Pandiscio, Bill Loccisano, Charles Miers, Dung Ngo, Kathleen Anderson, Jim Nelson, Michael Hainey, Sarah Goldstein, Adam Rapoport, Andy Comer, Hooman Majd, Gene Pressman, and Anne Kennedy.

First published in the United States of America in 2011 by
Rizzoli International Publications, Inc.
300 Park Avenue South
New York, NY 10010
www.rizzoliusa.com

ISBN-13: 978-0-8478-3547-8
Library of Congress Control Number: 2010942803
© 2011 Rizzoli International Publications, Inc.
Text © 2011 Glenn O'Brien
"Glenn O'Brien: A Portrait" © 2011 Jean-Philippe Delhomme
Illustrations © 2011 Jean-Philippe Delhomme

Some chapters herein contain material published in another form in *GQ, 10Man,* and the *Bergdorf Goodman* magazine, which are gratefully acknowledged.

Design: Pandiscio Co./Bill Loccisano
Editor: Dung Ngo
Production: Maria Pia Gramaglia

Printed and bound in the United States of America

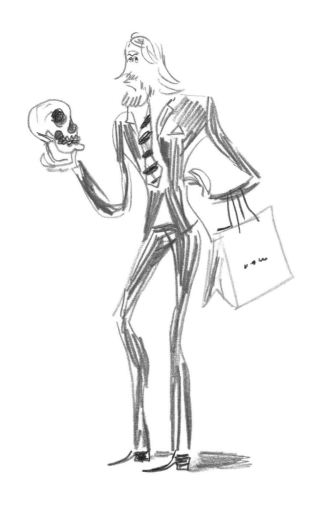

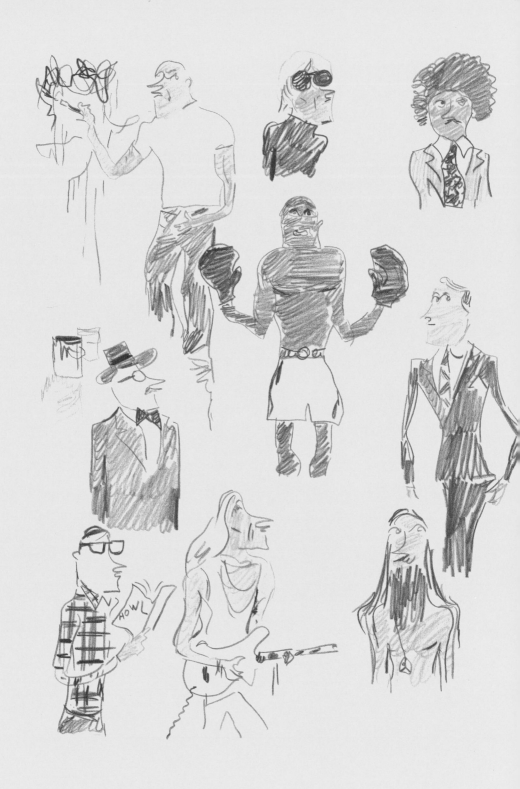